Guilherme Carlos Brech
Roberto Guarniero

Physiotherapy in Legg-Calvé-Perthes disease

CW00819970

Guilherme Carlos Brech
Roberto Guarniero

Physiotherapy in Legg-Calvé-Perthes disease

Conservative Treatments, Rehabilitation and Exercise

LAP LAMBERT Academic Publishing

Impressum/Imprint (nur für Deutschland/ only for Germany)

Bibliografische Information der Deutschen Nationalbibliothek: Die Deutsche Nationalbibliothek verzeichnet diese Publikation in der Deutschen Nationalbibliografie; detaillierte bibliografische Daten sind im Internet über http://dnb.d-nb.de abrufbar.
 Alle in diesem Buch genannten Marken und Produktnamen unterliegen warenzeichen-, marken- oder patentrechtlichem Schutz bzw. sind Warenzeichen oder eingetragene Warenzeichen der jeweiligen Inhaber. Die Wiedergabe von Marken, Produktnamen, Gebrauchsnamen, Handelsnamen, Warenbezeichnungen u.s.w. in diesem Werk berechtigt auch ohne besondere Kennzeichnung nicht zu der Annahme, dass solche Namen im Sinne der Warenzeichen- und Markenschutzgesetzgebung als frei zu betrachten wären und daher von jedermann benutzt werden dürften.

Coverbild: www.ingimage.com

Verlag: LAP LAMBERT Academic Publishing AG & Co. KG
Dudweiler Landstr. 99, 66123 Saarbrücken, Deutschland
Telefon +49 681 3720-310, Telefax +49 681 3720-3109
Email: info@lap-publishing.com

Herstellung in Deutschland:
Schaltungsdienst Lange o.H.G., Berlin
Books on Demand GmbH, Norderstedt
Reha GmbH, Saarbrücken
Amazon Distribution GmbH, Leipzig
ISBN: 978-3-8383-9755-9

Imprint (only for USA, GB)

Bibliographic information published by the Deutsche Nationalbibliothek: The Deutsche Nationalbibliothek lists this publication in the Deutsche Nationalbibliografie; detailed bibliographic data are available in the Internet at http://dnb.d-nb.de.
 Any brand names and product names mentioned in this book are subject to trademark, brand or patent protection and are trademarks or registered trademarks of their respective holders. The use of brand names, product names, common names, trade names, product descriptions etc. even without a particular marking in this works is in no way to be construed to mean that such names may be regarded as unrestricted in respect of trademark and brand protection legislation and could thus be used by anyone.

Cover image: www.ingimage.com

Publisher: LAP LAMBERT Academic Publishing AG & Co. KG
Dudweiler Landstr. 99, 66123 Saarbrücken, Germany
Phone +49 681 3720-310, Fax +49 681 3720-3109
Email: info@lap-publishing.com

Printed in the U.S.A.
Printed in the U.K. by (see last page)
ISBN: 978-3-8383-9755-9

I dedicate this book to my wife Tatiana and our daughter Gabriela, who are my inspiration in everything I do and every choice I make. I also dedicate this to my dad Peter and mom Maria Lúcia, who always supported me in every endeavor. They are the reason I am here at all, and made me who I am today.

I am heartily thankful to my supervisor, Roberto Guarniero, whose encouragement, guidance and support from the initial to the final level enabled me to develop an understanding of the subject. I am also thankful to Faculdade de Medicina da Universidade de São Paulo, represented by Professor Olavo Pires de Camargo, who encouraged and allowed me to write my dissertation in a book form.

Thiago thank you again for helping me with the translation!

Lastly, I offer my regards and blessings to all of those who supported me in any respect during the completion of the project.

Table of Contents

1. INTRODUCTION

This book deals with a relatively recently discovered disease that affects children. When treated as early as possible, these children can have a better quality of life. Until 1910, Legg-Calvé-Perthes disease (LCPD) had not been defined. Legg, in the United States of America, Calvé, in France, and Perthes, in Germany, conceptualized and described the disease around the same time (Nevelös, 1996). We believe this book's importance lies in the small quantity of scientific work studying the possible benefits of physical therapeutic treatment for this disease.

The incidence of LCPD has been found to vary according to the geographic location of evaluated groups. For instance, in Liverpool, England, 11.1 cases per 100,000 inhabitants were found and in Massachussetts, United States of America, the rate found was 5.1 children affected per 100,000 over the period of one year. On the other hand, in South Africa, the annual incidence found in Whites was 10.8 per 100,000 inhabitants, while in Blacks the rate was only .45 cases for every 100,000 inhabitants (Kealey et al., 2000). In the Chonnam province in Korea, the annual rate of occurrence of LCPD in children under 14 years of age was 3.7 per 100,000 inhabitants (Rowe et al., 2004). Unfortunately, in the literature reviewed, no information was found regarding the annual incidence of this disease in our country of Brazil.

LCPD is characterized by avascular necrosis of the ossification nucleus of the femur's proximal epiphysis, followed by subchondral fracture, revascularization and remodeling of the dead bone during the child's development (Figure 1 and 2).

The clinical picture is comprised of limping, pain, and limited articular range of motion (ROM) of the involved hip, especially abduction, extension, and medial rotation of the hip. The diagnosis is made according to the clinical picture and is confirmed by radiographic evaluation and complementary exams.

Treatment of LCPD has evolved since its first identification, and some controversy arose regarding the best form of treatment since their first descriptions (Meehan et al., 1992). The main goal of treatment is to retain the best morphology possible for hip articulation so as to avoid precocious degeneration and to maintain articular mobility while alleviating pain (Herring et al., 1993; Wang et al., 1995).

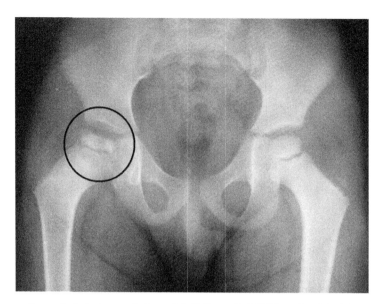

Figure 1. Anterior-posterior pelvic X-Ray with LCPD on the right hip.

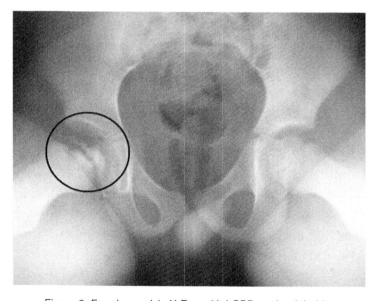

Figure 2. Frog Leg pelvic X-Ray with LCPD on the right hip.

Up to this moment, there is no consensus amongst professionals in the field regarding the best treatment for this disease. There are several conservative forms of treatment, and the earlier the patients are treated, the better the prognosis (Katz, 1967). Nevertheless, there are few studies that have evaluating the benefits of physical therapy in the treatment of LCPD as their goal. Most use physical therapy as a resource in combination with other treatments, but without directly evaluating its benefits (Herring et al., 2004a). Accordingly, while developing this study, no research was found that clearly defined the physical therapy exercises to be used and their real benefits.

This book was written based on a Master Degree Dissertation developed at the Faculdade de Medicina da Universidade de São Paulo in Brazil (Brech, 2006) and published as a scientific paper (Brech and Guarniero, 2006). The book has a detailed description of the general characteristics of patients with LCPD and also the actuation of the physiotherapy at the LCPD, described at the chapter of Literature Review.

Besides that, the book has a whole description of a study which aims was clinically evaluate from the possible effects of the physical therapy exercises proposed herein in comparison to the observational follow-up of patients with LCPD that is usually adopted.

This study has two hypotheses. The null hypothesis (H_0) being tested is the absence of a significant difference between the averages of the evaluated groups. The alternative hypothesis (H_A), meanwhile, is that there is a significant difference between the averages of those same groups.

2. LITARATURE REVIEW

The bibliographic review of published works was divided into the following:

2.1 General characteristics of Legg-Calvé-Perthes disease (LCPD)

2.2 Physiotherapy and Legg-Calvé-Perthes disease (LCPD)

2.1 General characteristics of LCPD

The literature review on the general characteristics of LCPD was based especially on work that discusses its clinical and radiographic aspects.

Catterall (1971) conducted a study with the goal of suggesting the degree of involvement of the proximal femoral epiphysis, determining a prognosis and an appropriate treatment. He studied 121 patients, totaling 133 hips. For four years or more, he observed 97 hips, 46 of which were not treated. He analyzed images of the femoral head with radiographs in the early stages and during the evolution of the disease. He classified the stages of LCPD into four types according to radiographic findings. In type I, patients have involvement of up to one quarter of the femoral head, which is limited to the anterior portion of the femoral head; in type II, the process involves the anterior half of the femoral head; in type III, two thirds of the bony nucleus is affected, and is radiographically denominated "head within a head;" and in type IV the entire epiphysis is affected. He also noted that the final outcome was not affected by treatment in children less than four years old. Female patients showed a worse prognosis. He described the radiographic signs of poor prognosis for the disease, such as the transradiant sign lateral to the physis ("Gage's sign"); lateral calcifications of the epiphysis; subluxation of the femoral head and flattening of the epiphyseal plate. He concluded that the prognosis varies according to the involvement of the epiphysis, that it is possible to classify the initial radiographs into four phases, that sex and age influence the final prognosis of the disease, and suggested that the signs of the head at risk be used in diagnosis.

Petrie and Bitenc (1971) conducted a study with 108 patients, and presented a new therapeutic method that allows for removing weight load during conservative treatment by restricting the hip. Up to that time, patients needed to be hospitalized for several months. The authors recommended a treatment using a plaster cast below the hips, keeping the hips in a position of abduction and medial rotation with the knee in extension, which allows not only for the flexion-extension of the hip joint, but for hip adductor tenotomy as well, if deemed necessary. Patients could then walk with the aid of crutches, and returned to their

8

school and social activities. The average length of immobilization was 19 months. The results obtained were good for 48.1% of patients, 16.7% were considered fair, and 35.2% were considered poor.

In 1978, Dickens and Menelaus applied Catterall's classification in order to assess its validity. Seventy patients with LCPD were studied retrospectively, clinically and radiographically. Hips were evaluated for range of movement (ROM); loss of muscle strength; difference in limb length and presence of Trendelenburg's sign. They rated a clinical outcome as "good" when the patient had no symptoms and had full hip ROM. The result was considered "fair" when the patient had no pain in the hip and presented little ROM restriction, especially medial rotation. Results were considered "poor" when the patients had both the symptom and ROM restriction.

Gershuni (1980) reported that a hip with severe impairment and joint incongruity, diagnosed radiologically, could present excellent ROM for the hip. However, a patient who presented very painful and marked hip ROM limitation could present less impairment radiographically.

In 1980, Mose reported the need to measure the femoral head lesion arising from LCPD in order to obtain a prognosis regarding osteoarthritis of the hip in adult patients. He demonstrated measurement of femoral head sphericity by means of concentric circles in two millimeter increments in anteroposterior and profile radiographs.

Catterall (1980) reported that 60% of patients did well without treatment, but that it was important to correlate his findings with other studies. According to the classification described by the author, indications for no treatment are Catterall patients classified as type I, II and III, aged less than five years, and having no signs of risk.

Edvardsen et al. (1981) clinically assessed their patients for the presence of pain, limping, Trendelenburg's sign, and measured the discrepancy in leg length and bilateral ROM.

In a study involving three medical centers, in 1981, Stulberg et al. created a radiological classification system based on results obtained after treatment of LCPD. This classification divided patients into five types: type I, normal femoral head; type II, rounded femoral head with shortened neck and enlarged metaphysis; type III, oval, not spherical, head; type IV, flattened head with short neck and deformed acetabular cavity; and type V, flat head with normal femoral neck and acetabular cavity.

9

In a multicenter study, Salter and Thompson (1984) analyzed the hips of 936 children with LCPD in 1122 radiographs and created a classification system divided into two types based on a radiographic indicator of subchondral lysis. Hips are considered type A when the extent of the lesion is up to half of the head. In type B, subchondral lysis has compromised more than half of the femoral head. They also concluded that the classification could only be used in the early stages of the disease, when the subchondral fracture is visible.

In 1992, Martinez et al. conducted a study of 31 patients (34 hips) with LCPD, Catterall classifications type III and IV, treated with abduction orthosis. They concluded that there is no indication for an orthosis for patients classified as type Catterall III and IV and/or Salter and Thompson type B.

Meehan et al. (1992) developed their own hip abduction orthosis, which is a modification of the orthosis developed by Petrie and Bitenc. Thirty-four patients with LCPD were studied and evaluated according to the Mose and Stulberg et al. classifications, as well as the criteria of the Pediatric Society of North America. According to the assessment, the use of orthosis did not show advantages over other methods of treatment. The abduction orthosis was very popular in the 1970s, but began to show poor results when patients were followed for long periods, through retrospective studies.

Herring et al. (1992) described a classification system based on the lateral pillar height of the epiphysis in the fragmentation phase, subdividing the hips into three types. Type A includes hips in which there is preservation of the lateral pillar or where there is a minimal reduction of its height. Type B are those with up to 50% of lateral pillar height of the epiphysis compromised. And in type C, there is greater than 50% reduction of lateral pillar height of the hips affected.

Yrjönen (1992) studied 80 hips treated with a Thomas splint and another 26 hips treated with bed rest. Clinical and radiographic evaluations were performed after an average of 35 years (28-47 years) after diagnosis. Osteoarthritis was found in 51 of the 106 hips treated, 15 of them in serious condition. Only 22 hips were classified as "good."

Tsao et al. (1997) reviewed 44 patients with LCPD. Patients were examined clinically 4.4 years, on average, after completion of treatment and imaging tests (bone scan and x-rays) were performed. Physical examination was correlated with the imaging findings. Upon physical examination, the mean ROM in the affected hip was 37° abduction, 119° of flexion, -5° extension, 14° of medial rotation and 30° lateral rotation. It was concluded that bone scintigraphy could be used to better determine the prognosis at disease onset, compared with the radiographs, thus enabling early intervention.

In 1998, Guille et al. studied 575 patients with LCPD and proposed that clinical evaluations should be based on goniometry. Affected hips without restrictions in ROM were considered a good result. Patients with few restrictions in ROM in the affected hip attained fair results, while patients with many limitations in the ROM of the affected hip achieved poor results.

Weinstein (2000) published the results of an extensive review of articles related to his clinical experience in pediatric orthopedics. He cited his study of 31 patients with LCPD (33 hips) classified as Catterall types III and IV who were treated with abduction orthosis. The average initial age of the patients was six years, and they were followed for seven years. Under criteria defined by Mose, no hip was rated "good." Twelve (35%) were classified as "fair" hips, and 22 hips (65%) were "poor." Based on these results, the author did not recommend the use of abduction orthoses for patients with LCPD classified as Catterall types III and IV.

In 2002, Gigante et al. compared the prognostic value of radiographic classifications of Catterall and Herring et al. in 32 patients with LCPD. All had unilateral involvement and had been treated with surgery. Using the radiographic classification of Stulberg et al., all cases were reevaluated at skeletal maturity. They noted that Catterall classification did not result in a meaningful prognosis during the final evaluation, except in some cases with signs of a "head at risk," such as lateral epiphyseal calcification and subluxation greater than four millimeters. The radiographic classification of Herring et al. showed better correlation with a prognosis when monitoring the disease. Younger age was reported to be one of the main predictors of a good prognosis, and patients with less than six years of age progressed very well, even when presenting with Herring et al. type C.

Lecuire (2002) studied 57 patients (60 hips) with LCPD, an average of 34 years after diagnosis of the disease. Among these, 48 patients (51 hips) were evaluated after a mean follow-up period of 50.2 years after disease onset. All patients had been treated the same way and admitted with or without skin traction for bed rest. The mean hospitalization time was 21 months. Pain, limping, ROM limitation, discrepancy in the length of legs and loss of muscle strength were clinically evaluated. Were evaluated radiographically according to the Mose classification. After 34 years of follow-up of 60 hips, 17 had moderate discomfort and 10 had strong discomfort. Among the patients followed for 50.2 years, 12 had undergone total hip arthroplasty and only 21 patients did not experience pain.

Laredo Filho et al. (2002) conducted a literature review of LCPD and described the clinical picture of the child with a limp and/or antalgic gate, with or without a history of previous trauma, with pain localized in the inguinal region or in the anteromedial portion of the thigh and knee. Because of the limitation of the ROM of the hip in all directions, primarily affecting medial rotation and abduction movements, disuse of the limb may result in atrophy of the thigh.

In 2003, Joseph et al. analyzed the results of 97 patients with LCPD, during a period of 25 years, who underwent varus osteotomy. Radiographs were evaluated by Mose classification in order to assess the appropriate moment to recommend surgery. They concluded that patients should be operated early, while still at the necrosis or fragmentation stage.

Grzegorzewshi et al. (2003) evaluated the hips of 197 patients with LCPD with unilateral involvement. Of these, 142 hips pertained to a type B Herring classification and 55 hips to a type C. All had radiographic examinations performed at four different times: at diagnosis, in the period that had the highest deformity in the sphericity ratio, after treatment was completed, and skeletal maturity. The treatment goal was to contain the femoral head. Seventy-four patients were treated conservatively with rest and skin traction in abduction, 21 patients with a cast, 74 with abduction orthosis and 26 patients with pelvic or femoral osteotomy. There was no significant difference in the final results of the different types of treatment.

Fabry et al. (2003) conducted a meta-analysis of the literature, showing that not all children under five years of age have a good treatment outcome. Children with little involvement and early-stage LCPD have demonstrated a better prognosis than children with more serious involvement of the femoral head and in later stages of the disease. Children with LCPD under five years of age are not exempt from presenting serious impairment in the hip. They concluded that younger children have greater chances of obtaining a better result than the older children, but results are not always good. Children over nine years of age almost always develop poorly.

According to Jacobs et al. (2004), the main goal of treatment of LCPD is to prevent hip deformities or incongruities, as well as to delay the development of a degenerative process in the hip joint in adulthood. Forty-three patients with unilateral disease LCPD were studied, presenting a Catterall classification type III or IV and Herring type B or C, treated with shelf acetabuloplasty. Patients were evaluated radiographically and data from their clinical history were collected. Clinical history included the time of the onset of symptoms and reports of pain. Pre- and post-operative physical examination were conducted to measure the ROM of the hip. The mean postoperative follow-up period was 3.7 years. Six patients continued having pain after surgery, while pre-operatively 21 patients reported having severe pain. All patients had no restrictions on their activities. There was a gain in ROM of the hip, medial rotation increased from 14° to 33.9° on average, and 14 patients showed an average discrepancy of 4.2 mm in lower limb length. The authors believed that shelf acetabuloplasty is a surgical procedure that is suitable for children over five years of age with severe LCPD.

According to Segev et al. (2004), conservative treatment does not affect the changing shape of the femoral head or joint congruity. Sixteen patients with severe LCPD were studied, all with severe pain and limitation of hip ROM, and having had hip arthrodiastisis. After arthrodiastisis surgery, all patients increased hip ROM by an average of 20° of flexion, 16° of abduction and 17° of medial rotation. All patients were able to walk without aids and Trendelenburg's sign disappeared in eight patients.

Agus et al. (2004) studied the reliability of inter and intra-observer Catterall, Salter-Thompson, Herring and Stulberg radiographic classifications in relation to the stage of treatment of LCPD. Both the Catterall and Salter-Thompson classification have good interrater reliability and intra-observer. The Stulberg classification obtained better results and more inter- and intra-observer reliability when used at least five years after completion of treatment. They concluded that the Catterall and Salter-Thompson classifications should be used to determine the treatment to be performed, and the Stulberg classification to rate the effectiveness of treatment of patients at skeletal maturity. They reported that doubts remained about the classification to be adopted to evaluate patients during the treatment period, and that there was a need to create a new, more reliable classification to be used during treatment.

Sugimoto el at. (2004) conducted a study of 56 patients with unilateral LCPD, using a new classification system. This system combined the classification of the posterior and lateral pillar of the femoral head to determine their correlation with prognosis of treatment. They found that flexion contractures and hip abduction can have a large effect on the posterior pillar classifications based on lateral radiographs, making separate left and right radiographic films necessary for symmetrical comparison.

Wiig et al. (2004) prospectively evaluated subchondral fractures as a predictor of the extent of necrosis of the femoral head. Over five years, 28 hospitals in 19 countries reported 392 new cases of LCPD. At the time of diagnosis, 92 patients (23.5%) had a subchondral fracture. They concluded that subchondral fracture is an early radiographic sign of LCPD, and is a sign for diagnosis and prognosis.

As part of a multicenter study, with the goal of rating the inter and intra-observer reliability of the lateral pillar and Stulberg classification of 345 hips, Herring et al. introduced a new type of lateral pillar classification: type B/C. This type is characterized by thin ossification and a 50% reduction of the original height of the lateral pillar. They concluded that these classifications have statistically significant inter-and intra-observer reliability. The modification of the lateral pillar classification and a redefinition of the Stulberg classification are sufficiently reliable and accurate for use in LCPD (Herring et al., 2004a).

According Erkula et al. (2004), one of the most important etiological factors for the development of osteoarthritis is LCPD.

Rowe et al. (2004) put forward that deformity of the femoral head due to LCPD may cause subsequent osteoarthritis of the hip. An experimental study in rabbits was conducted in which they were grouped according to three criteria: devascularization and immobilization combined, devascularization, and immobilization. In the pathophysiology of femoral head subluxation, initially, necrosis and a repair process occur. Next, subluxation generates an abnormal distribution of pressure on the acetabulum over the femoral head's softened articular surface. Finally, abnormal acetabular articular pressure on the femoral head causes deformities in the femoral head. They concluded that subluxation of the femoral head with avascular necrosis in adult rabbits results in a higher incidence of deformities and stress on the femoral head.

Grzegorzewski et al. (2005) conducted a study involving 261 patients with unilateral LCPD and determined factors in the disease that create a length discrepancy in the legs. All hips were treated with femoral head containment methods: bed rest with skin traction in abduction, Petrie cast, plaster cast, varus osteotomy, Salter osteotomy and shelf acetabuloplasty. According to the authors, the discrepancy in leg length is unrelated to age at the onset of symptoms or to the treatment adopted, whether surgical or conservative, since age at the onset of symptoms does not always coincide with the onset of the disease. However, leg length discrepancy is related to the onset of the disease and may result in a shorter limb.

According to Kitakoji et al. (2005), the residual clinical problems associated with any surgical procedure are pain, limitation of ROM of the hip, difference in length of the lower limbs, insufficient abductor musculature, and post-surgical scarring. At the end of skeletal

14

maturity, of the patients with LCPD who had undergone a varus or Salter osteotomy, some had a restricted hip ROM, with a difference of 10° of abduction and 30° of hip flexion between the affected side compared and the uninvolved side. The authors concluded that conservative treatments are also effective for treating the disease, and that surgical treatments are not always preferable to conservative treatments. One advantage of surgical LCPD treatment is the shorter time of inconvenience to the patient. The Salter osteotomy is the most often recommended.

Guarniero et al. (2005) conducted a retrospective study in which they evaluated the clinical and radiographic data of 67 patients with LCPD described in medical records. They found an average hip ROM of 102.2° of flexion, 28° of abduction, medial rotation of 15.4° and 30° of lateral rotation. The authors believed that muscle function tests should be part of the initial evaluation of patients with LCPD in order to compare the degree of muscle strength of the involved limb with that of the uninvolved limb. They concluded that the clinical picture is well defined, presenting pain, limping and decreased ROM of the hip, especially flexion, abduction and medial rotation.

2.2 Physiotherapy and LCPD

The literature review on physiotherapy and LCPD was based on studies addressing its role with the disease.

In a literature review, Carpenter (1975) reported that little had been written about the contribution of bed rest with skin traction, in combination with physiotherapy, to a decrease in muscle spasms, pain, or a gain of ROM in patients with LCPD. The author describes the physical therapy techniques used in the Scottish Rite Hospital (Dallas, USA), associated with rest and skin traction:

- Assisted active, active and active-resistance exercises in all planes, with emphasis on extension, abduction and medial rotation to maintain muscle tone, mobility and prevent muscle atrophy;

- Active exercise with all limbs during treatment in a Hubbard tank with warm water to decrease spasms, and exercises that help to prevent reductions in muscle tone;

- Proprioceptive neuromuscular facilitation, using bilateral and reciprocal patterns;

- Cryotherapy for reducing muscle spasms before exercises, when necessary.

Carpenter also emphasized the need to regularly measure hip ROM. He said exercises should be started on the day a framework is created for patients, and should be done until the full ROM of the hip is achieved. He concluded that physical therapists could help orthopedic surgeons in the treatment of LCPD, relieving pain and improving ROM of the hip.

In 1980, Jani and Dick conducted a retrospective study of three groups of patients with LCPD, divided according to the proposed treatment. In one of the groups, physical therapy was performed for one or two weeks, followed by varus osteotomy, and physiotherapy again for three to six months after surgery. Results for this group were excellent, and the authors questioned whether it was necessary to carry out a surgical procedure, or whether these patients would have scored well with only conservative treatment.

Klisic et al. (1980) advocated early hip joint exercises and continuing them until the lesion had completed regeneration.

Bowen et al. (1982) analyzed 392 patients (430 hips) with LCPD who had been treated by different surgical and conservative procedures at the Alfred I. duPont Institute (Wilmington, Delaware, USA). They evaluated radiographic exams and data from medical records. They noted that nine patients were treated with skin traction, in combination with physical therapy sessions, until reaching total hip ROM. The also described that the increased growth of the greater trochanter caused a deficiency in hip abductor muscles, and that this deficiency could be treated with muscle strengthening exercises, usually relieving fatigue due to hip pain.

Sposito et al. (1992) conducted a study with 28 patients with LCPD treated by modified Salter osteotomy, and clinically examined the patients at three stages: preoperative, postoperative and after rehabilitation. Clinical examination included analysis of the degree of joint dysfunction (goniometry and muscle function test) for all hip movements, dynamic assessment of joint dysfunction, evaluation of the discrepancy of limb length, assessing the degree of change in posture, and gait analysis. All patients were referred for physical therapy after surgery, however, only 15 patients actually completed it. The rehabilitation program consisted of kinesiotherapy with muscle strengthening and passive exercises, aimed at complete ROM of the affected hip. They concluded that with rehabilitation treatment the kinetic-postural picture tends to improve, especially in younger, male patients, and may have worse outcomes with no rehabilitative treatment.

16

Ishida et al. (1994) studied 16 patients with LCPD who underwent a Salter osteotomy with fixation by two or three threaded pins and without cast immobilization for the early physiotherapeutic setup. They concluded that no immobilization during the postoperative period made early physical therapy possible, allowing patients to more quickly return to their activities.

A review by Herring (1994) demonstrated the difficulty of comparing different types of LCPD treatment because of the diverse evaluation criteria used in the literature. Most studies suggest that patients with less than six years of age usually have a good treatment prognosis, regardless of the treatment proposed. The goals of treatment are a reduction of symptoms, containment of the femoral head and total recovery of ROM. Hip exercises were done to improve symptoms such as pain and decreased ROM as a function of muscle spasm, and the use of anti-inflammatories was suggested. The author concluded that controlled studies, which are actually very difficult to perform, were needed.

Guarniero et al. (1995) studied hip cheilectomies. Patients remained hospitalized for post-operative skin traction, balanced on the lower extremity, operated for two to three weeks, and to carry out physiotherapy exercises, particularly hip abduction. The follow-up period ranged from two months to four years and six months, with an average of one year and eight months. Sixteen of the patients presented pain complaints in pre-treatment. Eight progressed without pain after the operation, one patient still had pain during movement. In seven patients there was no change in the pain. There was an improvement in the average degree of flexion (20°), abduction (27.7°), lateral rotation (30°) and medial rotation (25°). Three patients showed no improvement in clinical status.

Wang et al. (1995) studied and compared five methods of treatment in 460 patients. To be included in the study, patients were clinically and radiographically diagnosed with LCPD, had reached skeletal maturity and had completed one of five treatments. Patients were divided into five groups according to the proposed treatment. In the Scottish Rite orthosis group with skin traction, patients had previously undergone physiotherapy to relieve pain, correct limping and the ROM limitation of the hip. In the weight-bearing restriction group, patients underwent intensive physical therapy with exercises for maintaining hip ROM. In the Petrie cast, varus osteotomy and Salter osteotomy groups, patients did not undergo any type of exercise. Patients were evaluated radiographically by Mose classification. In the Scottish Rite orthosis group, 20 of 41 hips (49%) studied were considered satisfactory and the others unsatisfactory. In the weight-bearing restriction and physical therapy group, 20 of 41 hips (49%) studied were considered satisfactory and the others unsatisfactory. In the Petrie brace group, 18 of 29 hips (62%) studied were considered satisfactory, and others unsatisfactory. In the varus osteotomy group, nine of 15 hips (60%) studied were considered satisfactory, the others unsatisfactory. In the Salter osteotomy group, nine of 15 hips (60%) studied were considered satisfactory and other unsatisfactory. They concluded that the results did not determine the best treatment for LCPD, treatment recommendations should take into account the patient's social condition, and that the Scottish Rite orthosis was not found to be as promising as had been previously described in the literature.

At two medical centers in Japan, patients with LCPD were assessed by radiographs two years after treatment had ended. At the medical center for children in Shiga, of the 118 patients who were treated from 1980 to 1991, 98 patients used a unilateral brace with 30° of flexion, abduction and external rotation. Parents were instructed to perform daily exercises for the affected hip with the children so as to prevent joint contracture. In the general hospital in Kobe, of the 125 patients treated from 1971 to 1991, 110 patients were treated with the modified Petrie cast. The bars of the cast was removed twice a day to perform passive exercises. Of the patients who were treated by the unilateral brace, 11 patients (11.2%) had bilateral involvement and four patients (4.1%) had been diagnosed with bilateral involvement before the beginning of treatment. In six patients (6.1%), contralateral hip was affected during treatment after an average of 15 months. Of the patients who were treated with the modified Petrie cast, five (4.5%) had bilateral involvement before treatment, but no other child developed the disease in the contralateral hip during the use of this device (Futami and Suzuki, 1997).

Wall (1999), in his review study, reported that etiology, prognosis and early treatment remain an enigma for the orthopedist. He made recommendations for treatment, among them, that when symptoms appear, bed rest, skin traction and physiotherapy exercises for stretching are recommended.

Keret et al. (2002), in a case study, restricted weight-bearing to relieve pain and prevent the limitation of the hip ROM, without success. However, physical therapy, in combination with the use of NSAIDs, achieved some improvement. Physiotherapy exercises were done on the ground and in water, thereby maintaining good ROM of the hip.

According to Schmid et al. (2003), patients with decreased ROM should perform physical therapy before undergoing surgical procedures such as varus osteotomy.

Wild et al. (2003) evaluated 87 patients with LCPD and 54 patients (59 hips) were included in the study for having had X-ray examinations during the reossification phase. The aim of this study was to evaluate the risk of patients developing osteoarthritis secondary to the disease. Thus, patients were evaluated at skeletal maturity and after having undergone conservative treatment. Age ranged from 18 to 50 years, and the average time between treatment of the disease and the reevaluation was 26 (15 to 45) years. Patients were divided into two groups: Thomas splint or plaster cast (32 hips), and observation or rehabilitation (27 hips). After evaluation, all patients had pain and hip ROM limitation, and 50% had walking limitation. Patients were divided by Catterall classification, irrespective of treatment: group A (Catterall types I and II) and group B (Catterall types III and IV). In group A, of 29 hips, six had little osteoarthritis and one hip had grade two osteoarthritis. In group B, of 30 hips, all had osteoarthritis, six hips had grade one, 13 had grade two, 11 had grade three and two had already undergone total hip arthroplasty. Groups were compared according to treatment performed. In group A's patients (29 hips), of the 12 hips that were treated with a Thomas splint or plaster cast, one had osteoarthritis, whereas of the 17 hips treated with observation or rehabilitation, eight showed some degree of osteoarthritis. In group B's patients (30 hips), all 20 hips that were treated with a Thomas splint or plaster cast as well as the 17 hips that were treated with observation or rehabilitation had osteoarthritis. The authors reported that maintaining free ROM is important to maintaining joint congruence, and that physiotherapy is needed to maintain mobility. Studies to evaluate the effects of physiotherapy in LCPD, however, are not found in literature. They concluded that treatment should seek the centralization of the femoral head and, to prevent deformities, one must combine the use of orthesis with physical therapy sessions.

When there is a decrease of hip ROM, physical therapy exercises, in combination with skin traction, before or during the use of an abduction brace is recommended (Aksoy et al., 2004).

Herring et al. (2004b) conducted a multicenter study with 438 patients (451 hips) in which each researcher performed the same type of treatment for each patient. The five treatments performed were 1) observation with restricted physical activities, 2) brace, 3) exercises to gain hip ROM, 4) femoral osteotomy, and 5) innominate osteotomy. Ages ranged from 6 to12 years and no patient had any other type of treatment before the study. Of all patients, 337 (345 hips) were followed until skeletal maturity, classified by the modified Herring classification and the Stulberg classification. In the group that performed exercises to gain hip ROM, patients were instructed to perform an exercise program for stretching the adductors and active exercises to gain hip ROM, at least once a day. Initially, assisted active exercises with emphasis on hip abduction were performed. If the loss of hip ROM persisted, skin traction was performed. If the restrictions persisted further, patients could use abduction bracing for up to six weeks. No statistical difference between groups for the treatments were found. They concluded that lateral pillar classification and age at disease onset is strongly correlated with the outcomes of patients with LCPD. Patients with more than eight years of age and lateral pillar B or B/C have better results with surgery. In lateral pillar type B, patients with less than eight years of age have more favorable outcome, regardless of treatment. Patients of type C lateral pillar, of all ages, often have poor outcomes regardless of treatment.

Carney and Minter (2004) retrospectively studied the effectiveness of a non-surgical program to gain passive ROM in patients with LCPD. From April 1990 until February 1999, they evaluated 335 patients with LCPD. During the same period, 118 patients were diagnosed with LCPD and treated non-surgically to achieve full ROM of hip abduction. The study included 74 patients with unilateral LCPD. Medical records and radiograph data were reviewed. Nonsurgical treatments performed were bed rest, skin traction with progressive bilateral hip abduction, physical therapy with bicycle and hydrotherapy. Forty-two patients reached $30°$ or more of abduction with hip extension. Thus, they concluded that non-surgical treatment can be used to gain ROM in the hip.

In a prospective controlled study with preliminary results, Maxwell et al. (2004) compared arthrodiastasis in 15 hips with treatments described in the literature performed on 30 hips. After the removal of external fixation, two patients were required to perform a manipulation under anesthesia and physical therapy because of stiffness. They reported that the best treatment still remains unclear. Patients will be followed until skeletal maturity to achieve more expressive results, although preliminary results have shown considerable potential.

Westhoff et al. (2004) conducted a study involving 33 patients with unilateral LCPD. An evaluation using the three-dimensional motion analysis system (VICON 512) was conducted. Patients walked in order to evaluate the transfer of weight from one limb to the contralateral limb, evaluating the kinetic parameters of the hip in the frontal plane. The data were compared with those of normal children. Two movement disorders were detected. Three patients had a thoracic inclination toward the affected side for less than two seconds, a tilt of the pelvis to the unaffected side for over two seconds and an adduction of the hip for more than two seconds. In the other pathological movement, 12

20

patients showed a thoracic tilt toward the affected side for less than two seconds, a pelvic tilt for less than a second and a hip adduction for less than a second. According to the authors, there were deviations in the frontal plane when the patients with LCPD walked. The movement patterns should be trained and treated by physiotherapy, since they are detrimental to the joint.

Roy (2005) conducted a study of nine patients with hip pain, who had LCPD in childhood, and eight having had previous surgeries. All patients had discomfort or symptoms that influenced daily activities, and had not achieved relief with medication and three months of physical therapy. Eight hips had intra-articular abnormalities. Seven showed improvement after arthroscopy and resumed their activities, even sports. Three patients required a surgical procedure.

A patient with LCPD underwent hip arthrodiastasis and a physical therapy program. The patient was monitored twice a week for seven months, five months with the arthrodistractor device. Physical therapy consisted of exercises to gain ROM and muscle function. The patient was assessed by goniometry in three stages: before installing the arthrodistractor, two weeks after installing the unit, and eight weeks after its removal. The muscle function test was performed two weeks and eight weeks after withdrawal of arthrodistractor. The results show a significant improvement in ROM of the hip and in knee muscle function of the affected limb with physical therapy, suggesting that it may play a role in functional recovery of children with LCPD undergoing arthrodistractor installation (Felicio et al., 2005).

3. STUDY METHODS

3.1 Subjects

20 patients, of both sexes, with LCPS were the subjects for this study, evaluated from November 2003 to September 2005 at the Group of Pediatric Orthopaedics, from the Institute of Orthopedics and Traumatology, at the Hospital das Clínicas da Faculdade de Medicina da Universidade de São Paulo (IOT/HC-FMUSP) - Brazil. Guardians signed Hospital das Clínicas da Universidade de São Paulo informed consent forms, which were approved by the ethics committee (research protocol 680/03) and were informed of all of the steps involved in the study. After radiographic evaluation of the hip and having fulfilled the criteria for inclusion, the patients were divided into two groups, A and B.

The inclusion criteria were the following:

- Confirmed diagnosis of unilateral Legg-Calvé-Perthes disease
- Absence of any other related injury of the hip
- Patients have not undergone any hip surgery
- Patients must not be on any medication that compromises the joint involved
- No patients with a neurologic disturbance accompanied by cognitive changes
- Conservative treatment is recommended
- Group B patients must be able to visit the IOT/HC-FMUSP twice a week for physical therapy sessions.

Exclusion criteria:

- Patient failed to show up for treatment
- Patient did not make himself/herself available for reevaluation
- Parient began to take medication that could affect the joint involved
- Any injury to the lower body that would limit the child's ability to execute any of the proposed exercises
- Presence of pain that would impede the execution of any of the exercises
- More than two consecutive absences from treatment

3.1.1 Study of the sample

Group A had 10 patients and Group B also had 10. Two patients from Group B were excluded, as was one from Group A.

Descriptive statistics were calculated for the age of the patients, displayed as group statistics (Table 1) and graphed as values for each age (Figure 3). The mean age for the two groups was compared using a Student's t-test.

Table 1 – Descriptive statistics for patients' age (years), according to the assigned group included in the study.

Group	Number of cases	Mean	Standard deviation	Minimum	Median	Maximum
A	9	5,6	1,4	3,3	6,0	7,5
B	8	5,7	1,3	3,5	5,5	7,4

$p= 0. 956$, i.e. the mean ages are the same.

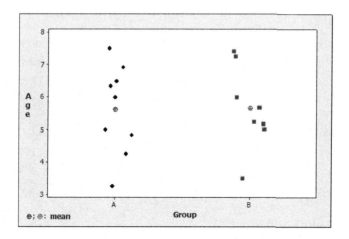

Figure 3 – Individual and mean values for age (years) in groups A and B

For sex, race, hip affected, dominant side, Catterall classification, Herring et al. Classification, and Salter-Thompson classification, incidence was calculated for each category in each group. The incidence of the radiographic classifications were represented in bar graphs (Figure 4).

Each category's probability of occurrence in the population was compared using the probability ratio test.

➢ Sex

In Group A, 11.1% of the patients were female, and in Group B, 12.5%. There is no significant difference between the percentages of males and females in the two groups (p=1.000).

➢ Race

In Group A, 77.8% of the patients were Caucasian, 22.2% were Black, and in Group B, these percentages were 87.5% and 12.5%, respectively. The incidence of Caucasian and Black races in the two populations are statistically equal (p= 0.596).

➢ Hip affected

In Group A, 33.3% of the patients had the right hip affected, 66.7% the left. In Group B, these percentages are 75% and 25%, respectively. No statistically significant difference between the two groups was detected in relation to these incidences (p=0.081).

➢ Dominance

55.6% of the patients in Group A and 75% of patients in Group B were right side dominant. No significant difference was detected between the incidences of the two groups (p = 0.620). There was no evidence of a relationship between dominant side and hip affected in either group (p=1.000).

➢ Catterall Classification

77.8% of the patients in Group A were classified as type II, and 22.2% were type III. In Group B, 25% were type I, 50% were type II, and 25% were type III. The hypothesis of equal Catterall distribution between the two groups was not rejected (p=0.170).

➢ Herring Classification

In Group A, 22.2% of the cases presented type A, and 77.8% presented type B. In Group B, 37.5% presented type A, while 62.5% presented type B (p= 0.490).

➢ Salter-Thompson Classification

44.4% of the patients presented type A in Group A, 37.5% in Group B. The rest of the patients could not be classified (NDA).

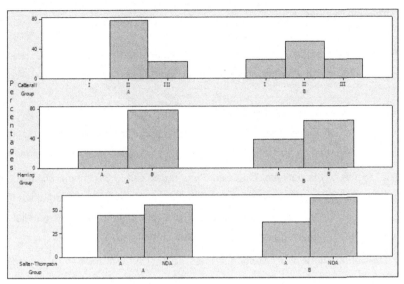

Figure 4 – Variable percentages for radiographic classifications, divided into Groups A and B

3.2 Type of study

Nonrandomized prospective controlled study, in which patients were divided into two groups and followed two different treatments. Groups were defined according to the availability of the patients and their guardians. Patients who could visit the Institute twice a week for 12 weeks were included in group B. For group A, observational accompaniment was done for 12 weeks without treatment. Group B underwent physical therapy twice a week for 12 weeks. In both groups, guardians were instructed to ensure the children did not engage in any physical activity that would impact the acetabulofemoral joint.

3.2.1 Inclusion criteria

The following personal data were collected from both groups at the beginning of the study: complete name, address, date of birth, sex, race, contact telephone number, guardian identification information, hip affected and dominant side. A clinical evaluation was conducted on each patient.

3.2.1.1 Clinical evaluation

The physical therapist conducting the study evaluated the lower limbs of patients in both groups, before and after treatment, as described below:

Range of motion evaluation (Goniometry)

Hip range of motion was evaluated, including: flexion, extension, abduction, adduction, medial rotation and passive lateral rotation, using a Carci® goniometer.

The degree of the patients' hip flexion was measured in the supine position, flexing the hip to be measured, with the knee bent. The goniometer was positioned along the axis of movement of the hip being examined and one of its arms was set parallel to the contralateral limb, while the other followed the axis of the flexed limb.

To measure extension, patients laid in prone position with their limbs extended, the axis of the goniometer affixed to the joint in question, with the affixed arm parallel to the axis of the contralateral limb and the movable arm following the extending limb's displacement towards the extension.

To measure abduction, patients were placed in the prone position asked to abduct the limb to be measured. The goniometer was positioned with its fixed arm placed in a line determined by the anterior superior iliac spines and moving along the axis of the limb that is to move (Figure 5). The same positioning was use to measure the degree of adduction, asking the patient to adduct the limb in question.

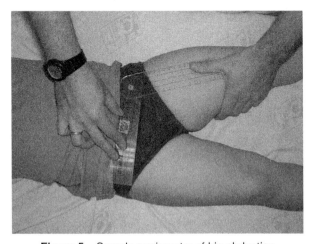

Figure 5 – Sample goniometry of hip abduction

Medial and lateral rotation was measured with patients seated, with knees bent at a 90° angle. The axis of the goniometer was positioned over the middle of the knee on the side to be measured, so that the fixed arm was parallel to the ground and the movable arm followed the axis of the tíbia in order to execute medial and lateral femoral rotations (Marques, 1997).

Evaluating degree of muscular strength

Hoppenfeld's (1999) criteria were adopted to evaluate the strength of the hip region. The strength of the affected side was compared to that of the unaffected side. Zero points were awarded when no muscular contraction was felt; one point was awarded when muscular contraction was felt but without producing movement in the joint; two points were awarded when movement was only produced towards the force of gravity; three points were awarded when the muscle contracted and moved against the force of gravity, but supporting little counter-resistance; and five points were awarded when movement against the force of gravity, with additional resistance, was normal.

Muscular strength measurement was completed for flexion, extension, abduction, adduction, medial and lateral rotation of the hips in the positions recommended by Kendall et al. (1995).

To evaluate hip flexor muscles with emphasis on the iliopsoas, patients remained supine with both legs extended. Patients were asked to flex the hip of the limb being evaluated, with the examiner stabilizing the opposing iliac crest.

The hip extensor muscles, especially the gluteus maximus, were evaluated with patients in prone position with knees flexed at 90 degrees, the examiner stabilizing the lumbar spine. Patients were asked to extend the limb being evaluated.

For the abductor muscles, especially the gluteus medius and minimus, patients remained in lateral position with the limb in contact with the table in semiflexion and the limb being evaluated in extension. The examiner stabilized the pelvis, preventing forward or backward rolling.

Adductor muscles (pectineus, adductor magnus, gracilis, adductor brevis and adductor longus) were evaluated with patients in lateral position, with both knees extended. The examiner held the leg on top in abduction and requested adduction of the limb on the bottom in an upward direction, away from the table, without rotation, flexion or extension of the hip or tilting pelvis.

27

Medial rotator muscles of the hip (tensor fasciae latae, gluteus medius and gluteus minimus) were evaluated with patients sitting at the table with knees flexed at the edge of the table. The examiner stabilized the limb to prevent abduction or adduction of the hip, and with the other hand on the lateral side of the leg above the ankle, evaluated the effort needed to rotate the thigh laterally.

Lateral rotator muscles (piriformis, quadratus femoris, obturator internus, obturator externus, superior gemellus and inferior gemellus) were evaluated in the same way as the medial rotators, changing only the positioning of the examiner's hand on the patient's leg to the medial side above the ankle, evaluating the effort to rotate the thigh medially.

Degree of joint dysfunction evaluation

To evaluate the degree of joint dysfunction, values found in goniometric evaluation and muscle strength assessment were used. In the goniometric evaluation, one point was assigned for every 5° of difference from the pattern of the unaffected hip for each movement of the joint. Similarly, one point was assigned for each degree of discrepancy in muscle strength for the groups tested, when comparing the result with the unaffected side. Points were summed before and after treatment to compare the groups, such as described by Sposito et al. (1992).

Radiographs from the beginning and end of treatment were studied to assess radiographic changes.

3.2.2 Treatment

3.2.2.1 Group A

Patients in group A were monitored at the clinic of the Department of Pediatric Orthopaedics, without treatment, for a period of 12 weeks. Parents or guardians were instructed to keep the patients from engaging in physical activities that involved some degree of impact (Catterall, 1980).

3.2.2.2 Group B

The patients underwent a rehabilitation program consisting of hip balance training, muscle stretching and muscle strengthening exercises. Each session was one on one and lasted 30 minutes on average.

Table 2 – Proposed sequence of the physical therapy program for patients with LCPD, group B, for a period of 12 weeks

	Stretching 3 X 20 seconds	Isometrics 3 X 20 seconds	Balance with bipedal support	Concentrics 3 X 10 repetitions	Balance with unipedal support
Sessions					
1 -4	X	X			
5 -8	X	X	X		
9 -12	X		X	X	
13 -24	X			X	X

3.2.2.2.1 Muscle stretching exercises

Patients performed passive exercises to stretch the hip muscles involved. Stretching was performed three times for each exercise modality, each held for twenty seconds (Kisner and Colby, 1998; Bandy and Sanders, 2003). Muscles or muscle groups selected for elongation of the involved hip were hamstring and triceps surae, rectus femoris and iliopsoas, adductors, medial rotator and lateral rotators.

Stretching of the iliopsoas and femoral rectus muscles: each patient was positioned supine with the hip and opposite knee flexed toward the chest of the patient to stabilize the pelvis to prevent hyperlordosis. The physiotherapist performed the hip extension stretch and flexion of the knee simultaneously (Figure 6).

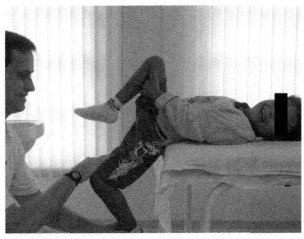

Figure 6 – Passive stretching of the iliopsoas and femoral rectus muscles

Stretching of the ischiotibial and triceps surae muscles: each patient was positioned supine with the knee extended and the opposite limb stabilized, and performed hip flexion with dorsiflexion of the ankle (Figure 7).

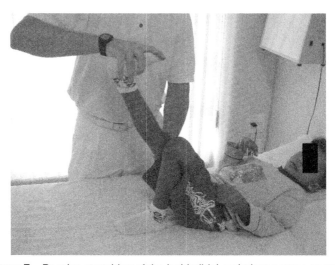

Figure 7 – Passive stretching of the ischiotibial and triceps surae muscles

Stretching of the hip abductor muscles: each patient was positioned supine with the knee of the opposite limb extended on the table. The therapist stabilized the hip side to be stretched and performed hip adduction with passive knee flexion (Figure 8).

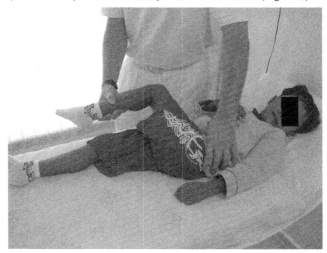

Figure 8 – Passive stretching of the hip abductor muscles

Stretching of the hip adductor muscles: each patient was positioned supine with knees in extension, stabilizing the pelvis, causing a pressure on the anterior iliac crest of the opposite side and keeping the opposite leg abducted. The physiotherapist abducted the stretched limb while maintaining the opposite limb static (Figure 9).

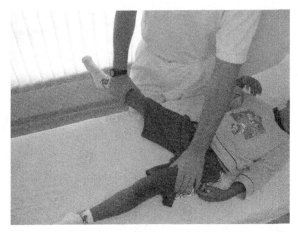

Figure 9 – Passive stretching of the hip adductor muscles

Stretching of the hip medial rotator muscles: Each patient was positioned prone, with hip extended and the knee of the stretched limb in 90º of flexion. The therapist stabilized the pelvis with one hand, pressing lightly on the buttocks with the other hand, holding the distal region of the tibia, rotating the hips laterally (Figure 10).

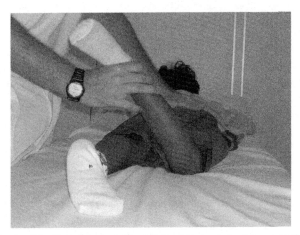

Figure 10 – Passive stretching of the hip medial rotator muscles

Stretching of the hip lateral rotator muscles: Each patient was positioned prone, with hip extended and the knee of the stretched limb in 90º of flexion. The therapist stabilized the pelvis with one hand, pressing lightly on the buttocks with the other hand, holding the distal region of the tibia, medially rotating the hip (Figure 11).

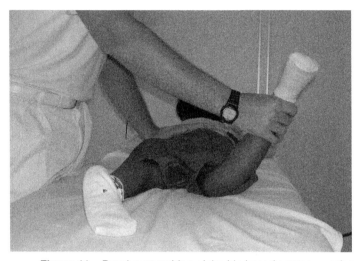

Figure 11 – Passive stretching of the hip lateral rotator muscles

3.2.2.2.2 Muscle strengthening exercises

Patients underwent exercises to strengthen the affected hip muscles. The strengthening exercises were performed three times for each exercise modality, maintaining isometric contractions for twenty seconds against gravity, until the eighth session. From the eighth session until the twenty-fourth session, isotonic concentric strengthening exercises were performed in three sets of ten repetitions each (Kisner and Colby, 1998; Bandy and Sanders, 2003; Felicio et al., 2005). Strengthening exercises such as isometric concentric exercises were performed in the same hip positions, such as Straight Leg Raise (SLR), i.e., muscle strengthening exercises for the involved hip flexors, extensors, hip abductors and adductors.

Strengthening of hip flexor muscles: each patient was positioned supine with knee extended. The knee and hip of the contralateral limb remained flexed, with the foot resting on the table. Patients performed flexion of the affected hip (Figure 12).

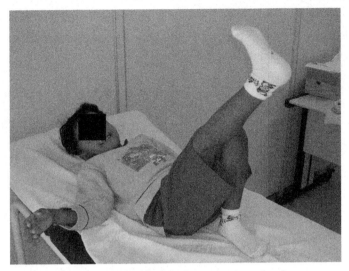

Figure 12 - Hip flexor muscle strengthening

Strengthening of hip extensor muscles: Each patient was positioned prone, with knees extended. The therapist stabilized the spine and the patient performed a hip extension (Figure 13).

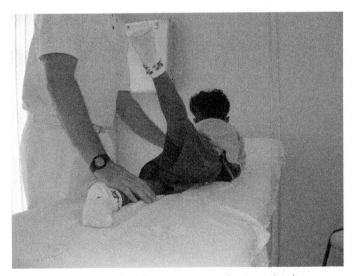

Figure 13 - Hip extensor muscle strengthening

Strengthening of hip abductor muscles: Each patient was positioned laterally with the limb to be strengthened at the top and the contralateral limb on the table with 90° flexion of the knee and hip. The physical therapist observed the lumbar spine to prevent patients from compensating while abducting the limb (Figure 14).

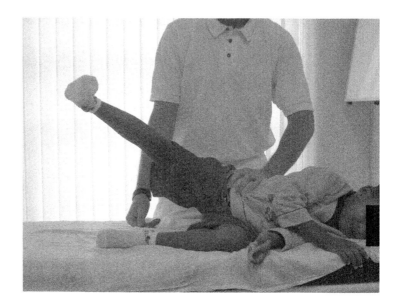

Figure 14 - Hip abductor muscle strengthening

Strengthening of hip adductor muscles: Each patient was positioned laterally on the side of the limb to be strengthened, aligned with the plane of the trunk. The contralateral limb was over the affected limb, with flexion, adduction and lateral rotation of hip and knee flexion with the foot flat on the table. Each patient performed a hip adduction with knee extension with bottom leg, and the therapist observed and corrected any lumbar spine compensation (Figure 15).

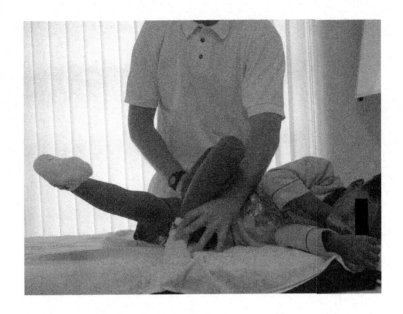

Figure 15 – Hip adductor muscle strengthening

3.2.2.2.3 Balance training

Balance training began in the fifth session. It was first performed on stable ground with stable bipedal support. Each patient was asked to remain in balance bipedally, with feet on the ground, without allowing any trunk displacement for as long as possible. When each patient could perform exercises on stable ground, in balance with bipedal support, exercises on unstable ground with bipedal support were begun. The resources used for unstable ground were, respectively: cushions, bidirectional balance board, and multidirectional balance board. From the thirteenth session onward, the patients began balancing on one foot, following the same sequence of stable and unstable ground (Bandy and Sanders, 2003; Westhoff et al., 2004) (Figure 16).

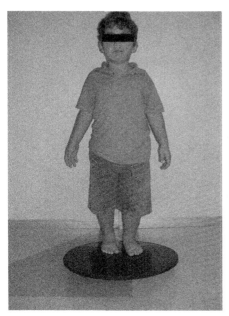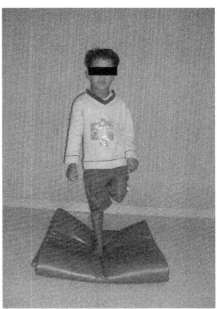

Figure 16 – Balance training on a multidirectional balance board with bipedal support, and on unstable ground, over a cushion with unipedal support

At the end of each therapy session, guardians were instructed to carry out some exercises at home on the days the patients did not have physical therapy treatment.

3.2.3 Statistical methods

It was performed descriptive analysis of the ADM ordinal quantitative parameters for flexion, extension, abduction, adduction, medial and lateral rotation of the hip according to the period (pre- and post-treatment), group (A and B), limb (affected and unaffected) and difference between subjects: case number (N), mean, standard deviation (SD), minimum, median and maximum pre- and post-treatment. Inference analysis was performed comparing the averages of each response with the two limbs, periods, and groups. In choosing the technique to be adopted, considered was given to the fact that the observation of both limbs and periods were done on the same individual. Since the comparison of the groups involved different individuals, repeated measures analysis of variance (Neter et al., 1996) was adopted. The assumptions for applying the technique were checked by the analysis of residuals. A significance level of ($p < 0.05$) was adopted. Differences between the two limbs were reviewed and the Bonferroni method applied to compare the mean differences in the following situations: pre- x post-treatment in Group A; pre- x post-treatment in Group B, Group A x Group B pre-treatment group; and Group A x Group B post-treatment.

For the inferential analysis of the degree of hip muscle strength, degrees were compared pre- and post-treatment. The McNemar test was adopted. This technique takes into account the scores observed in the same individual on two occasions. Comparisons were made separately for each group. A significance level of ($p < 0.05$) was adopted.

The degree of joint dysfunction classification was done through descriptive analysis of these ordinal quantitative parameters according to group and, secondly, the difference between groups: case number (N), mean, standard deviation (SD), minimum, median and maximum in the pre-and post-treatment periods. To assess the effect of group and period on the average level of articular dysfunction, repeated measures analysis of variance was used. Means were then compared in two by two using the Bonferroni method. A significance level of ($p < 0.05$) was adopted.

Descriptive analysis was done on patients' adherence to treatment in Group B for: number of cases (N), mean, standard deviation (SD), minimum, median and maximum.

Results were rounded scientifically and were presented to the two decimal places in tables and three decimal places or until the first significant digit in the statistical results.

In all analyses, the Minitab ® Statistical Software Release 14 (Copyright © 2005 Minitab Inc, State College, PA - USA) application was used.

4. STUDY RESULTS

4.1 Analysis of the range of motion of the hip

4.1.1 Descriptive analysis

Table 3 – Descriptive statistics for range of motion of hip flexion in affected and unaffected
limbs, and differences of flexion in the two limbs, pre- and post-treatment

Period	Limb	Group	N	Mean	SD	Minimum	Median	Maximum
Pre	Affected	A	9	116.67	7.50	105	120	130
		B	8	110.63	8.63	100	110	120
	Not Affected	A	9	122.22	7.12	110	120	135
		B	8	121.25	3.54	120	120	130
	Difference	A	9	5.56	6.35	0	5	15
		B	8	10.63	9.43	0	12.5	20
Post	Affected	A	9	115.56	8.82	100	120	130
		B	8	120	4.63	115	120	130
	Not Affected	A	9	122.22	7.12	110	120	135
		B	8	121.25	3.54	120	120	130
	Difference	A	9	6.67	7.5	0	5	20
		B	8	1.25	2.32	0	0	5

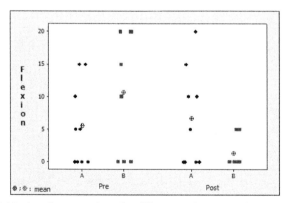

Figure 17 – Individual and mean values for differences in range of motion of hip flexion,
pre- and post-treatment

Table 4 – Descriptive statistics for range of motion of hip extension in the affected and unaffected limbs, and differences in the lengths of two limbs, pre and post-treatment

Period	Limb	Group	N	Mean	SD	Minimum	Median	Maximum
Pre	Affected	A	9	15.56	5.83	10	15	25
		B	8	10.63	4.17	5	10	20
	Not Affected	A	9	16.67	6.12	10	15	25
		B	8	13.13	4.58	10	10	20
	Difference	A	9	1.11	2.21	0	0	5
		B	8	2.50	3.78	0	0	10
Post	Affected	A	9	14.44	6.35	5	15	25
		B	8	13.13	4.58	10	10	20
	Not Affected	A	9	16.11	6.01	10	15	25
		B	8	13.75	5.18	10	10	20
	Difference	A	9	1.67	3.54	0	0	10
		B	8	0.63	1.77	0	0	5

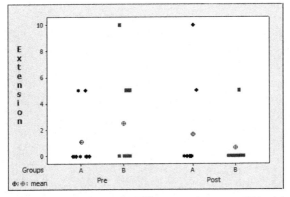

Figure 18 – Individual and mean values for differences in range of hip extension movement, pre- and post-treatment

Table 5 – Descriptive statistics for hip abduction range of movement in affected and unaffected limbs in the pre- and post-treatment periods

Period	Limb	Group	N	Mean	SD	Minimum	Median	Maximum
Pre	Affected	A	9	32.78	5.07	25	30	40
		B	8	25.0	5.98	15	27.5	30
	Not Affected	A	9	40.56	3.91	35	40	45
		B	8	38.75	5.18	30	40	45
	Difference	A	9	7.78	5.65	0	10	15
		B	8	13.75	7.44	0	15	25
Post	Affected	A	9	28.89	4.17	25	30	35
		B	8	36.25	7.44	25	40	45
	Not Affected	A	9	41.11	2.205	40	40	45
		B	8	40.63	3.2	35	40	45
	Difference	A	9	12.22	4.41	5	10	20
		B	8	4.38	5.63	0	2.5	15

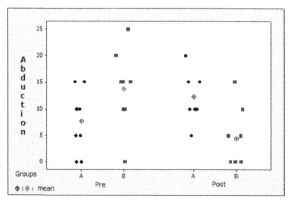

Figure 19 – Individual and mean values for differences in range of hip abduction movement, pre- and post-treatment

Table 6 – Descriptive statistics for hip adduction range of movement for affected and unaffected limbs, and adduction differences between the two limbs, in the pre- and post-treatment periods

Period	Limb	Group	N	Mean	SD	Minimum	Median	Maximum
Pre	Affected	A	9	21.11	6.01	15	20	30
		B	8	17.50	3.78	10	20	20
	Not Affected	A	9	25.00	6.12	15	30	30
		B	8	25.00	5.98	15	27.5	30
	Difference	A	9	3.89	5.46	0	0	15
		B	8	7.50	5.35	0	10	15
Post	Affected	A	9	16.67	5.59	10	20	25
		B	8	21.25	4.43	15	20	30
	Not Affected	A	9	24.44	5.83	15	25	30
		B	8	23.13	5.94	15	20	30
	Difference	A	9	7.78	7.55	0	5	20
		B	8	1.88	3.72	0	0	10

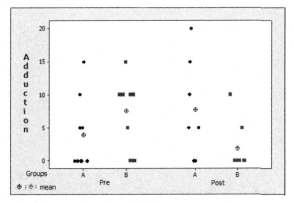

Figure 20 – Individual and mean values for differences in range of hip adduction movement, pre- and post-treatment

41

Table 7 –   Descriptive statistics for hip medial rotation range of movement for affected and
unaffected limbs, and medial rotation differences between the two limbs, in the
pre- and post-treatment periods

Period	Limb	Group	N	Mean	SD	Minimum	Median	Maximum
Pre	Affected	A	9	37.78	7.95	20	40	45
		B	8	28.75	8.35	20	30	40
	Not Affected	A	9	40.0	4.33	30	40	45
		B	8	40.63	4.96	30	40	45
	Difference	A	9	2.22	4.41	0	0	10
		B	8	11.88	6.51	0	10	20
Post	Affected	A	9	36.11	9.61	20	40	45
		B	8	38.75	5.82	30	40	45
	Not Affected	A	9	40	4.33	30	40	45
		B	8	40.63	4.96	30	40	45
	Difference	A	9	3.89	6.97	0	0	20
		B	8	1.88	3.72	0	0	10

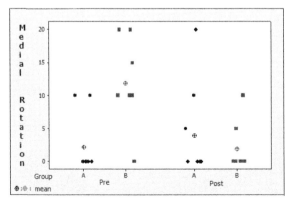

Figure 21 –   Individual and mean values for differences in range of hip medial rotation
movement, pre- and post-treatment

42

Table 8 – Descriptive statistics for hip lateral rotation range of movement for affected and unaffected limbs, and lateral rotation differences between the two limbs, in the pre- and post-treatment periods

Period	Limb	Group	N	Mean	SD	Minimum	Median	Maximum
Pre	Affected	A	9	36.67	7.07	25	40	45
		B	8	35.63	6.23	30	35	45
	Not Affected	A	9	40.00	6.12	25	40	45
		B	8	40.63	4.96	35	40	50
	Difference	A	9	3.33	5.59	0	0	15
		B	8	5.00	4.63	0	5	10
Post	Affected	A	9	34.44	6.82	25	35	45
		B	8	38.13	4.58	30	40	45
	Not Affected	A	9	40.00	6.12	25	40	45
		B	8	40.63	4.96	35	40	50
	Difference	A	9	5.56	6.35	0	5	15
		B	8	2.50	3.78	0	0	10

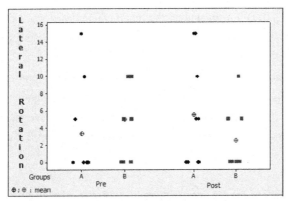

Figure 22 – Individual and mean values for differences in range of hip lateral rotation movement, pre- and post-treatment

4.1.3 Inferential analysis

- **Flexion:** There is no difference between the mean differences of flexion of the affected and unaffected limbs pre- and post-treatment in group A (p = 0.970). The average difference in the pre- period is greater than the post-treatment in group B (p <0.001). In the pre-treatment period, the differences are higher on average in group B than in group A (p = 0.010). Post-treatment, this relationship is reversed, and the mean difference in group B is smaller than in group A (p = 0.007).
- **Extension:** In group A, the mean differences in pre- and post-treatment are the same (p = 0.639). In group B, the average pre-treatment is higher than in post-treatment (p = 0.020). Pre-treatment, the mean difference in group B is higher than in group A (p = 0.072), and post-treatment, the means are the same in both groups (p = 0.236).
- **Abduction:** The differences were the same as in adduction. Group A has a higher mean difference in post-treatment (p = 0.005). Group B has a higher mean difference in pre-treatment (p <0.001), i.e. the differences between the two limbs decreases, on average, with treatment. In pre-treatment, group B has a higher average than group A (P <0.001). Post-treatment, the situation is reversed (p <0.001).
- **Adduction:** In group A, the mean difference post-treatment is higher than pre-treatment (p = 0.030). In group B, the average post-treatment is less than the pre-treatment (p = 0.002). In the pre-treatment, the average is higher in group B than in group A (p = 0.044). Post-treatment, group A has a higher mean difference (p = 0.002).
- **Medial rotation:** The mean differences between pre- and post-treatment are the same in group A (p = 0.350). In group B, the average is lower at post-treatment than at pre-treatment (p <0.001). Pre-treatment, the mean difference in group B is higher than in group A (p <0.001). Post-treatment, the average in group A and B are the same (p = 0.214).
- **Lateral rotation:** In group A, the mean differences are equal pre- and post-treatment (p = 0.051), and in group B the average post-treatment is less than the pre-treatment (p = 0.028). Pre-treatment, no difference was detected between the means of two groups (p = 0.167), and post-treatment, the average is lower in group B than in group A (p = 0.008).

Based on the above results, mean differences were recalculated when necessary and 95% confidence intervals were established. These results are presented in Table 9.

Table 9 – Means and confidence intervals with 95% confidence for differences between affected and unaffected limbs, divided by groups and periods

Variable	Group	Period	Mean	Confidence interval (95%)	
Flexion	A	Pre and Post	6.11	1.01	11.21
	B	Pre	10.63	2.75	18.50
		Post	1.25	-0.69	3.19
Extension	A	Pre and Post	1.02	-0.18	2.24
	B	Post			
	B	Pre	2.50	0.06	4.94 (*)
Adduction					
	A	Pre	3.89	-0.31	8.09
		Post	7.78	1.97	13.57
	B	Pre	7.50	3.03	11.97
		Post	1.88	-1.23	4.99
Abduction					
	A	Pre	7.78	3.43	12.12
		Post	12.22	8.83	15.61
	B	Pre	13.75	7.52	19.97
		Post	4.37	-1.23	4.98
Medial Rotation					
	A	Pre and Post	2.5	0.10	4.90
	B	Post			
	B	Pre	11.87	6.43	17.32
Lateral Rotation					
	A	Pre and Post	4.70	2.10	7.31
	B	Pre			
	B	Post	2.50	-0.66	5.66

(*) : 90% confidence coefficient

4.2 Analysis of degree of hip muscular strength

Table 10 – Distribution of frequencies and percentages of degree of hip flexion muscular strength in groups A and B, pre- and post-treatment

GROUP				Post 4	5	Total
A	Pre	4	Frequency	3		3
			%	100.00%		100.00%
		5	Frequency		6	6
			%		100.00%	100.00%
	TOTAL		Frequency	3	6	9
			%	33.30%	66.70%	100.00%
B	Pre	4	Frequency	1	5	6
			%	16.70%	83.30%	100.00%
		5	Frequency		2	2
			%		100.00%	100.00%
	TOTAL		Frequency	1	7	8
			%	12.50%	87.50%	100.00%

Group A: p= 1.000; Group B: p= 0.063

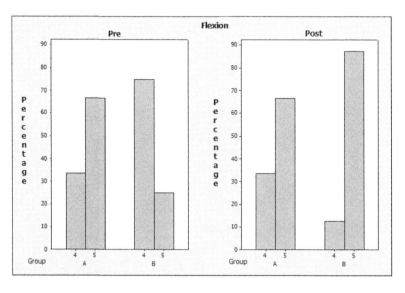

Figure 23 – Percentages for degree of hip flexion muscle strength in groups A and B, pre- and post-treatment

46

Table 11 – Distribution of frequencies and percentages of the degree of hip extension muscle strength in groups A and B, pre-and post-treatment

GROUP				Post 4	Post 5	Total
A	Pre	4	Frequency	5		5
			%	100.00%		100.00%
		5	Frequency	1	3	4
			%	25.00%	75.00%	100.00%
	TOTAL		Frequency	6	3	9
			%	66.70%	33.30%	100.00%
B	Pre	4	Frequency		2	2
			%		100.00%	100.00%
		5	Frequency		6	6
			%		100.00%	100.00%
	TOTAL		Frequency		8	8
			%		100.00%	100.00%

Group A: p= 1.000; Group B: p= 0.500

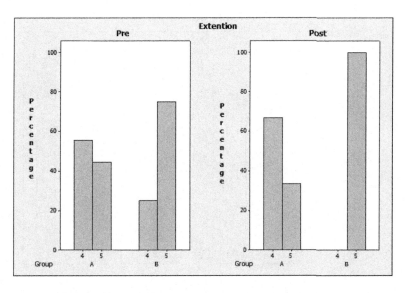

Figure 24 – Percentages for degree of hip extension muscle strength in groups A and B, pre- and post-treatment

Table 12 – Distribution of frequencies and percentages of the degree of hip abduction muscle strength in groups A and B, pre-and post-treatment

GROUP				Post 4	Post 5	Total
A	Pre	4	Frequency	2	1	3
			%	66.70%	33.30%	100.00%
		5	Frequency	1	5	6
			%	16.70%	83.30%	100.00%
	TOTAL		Frequency	3	6	9
			%	33.30%	66.70%	100.00%
B	Pre	4	Frequency		7	7
			%		100.00%	100.00%
		5	Frequency		1	1
			%		100.00%	100.00%
	TOTAL		Frequency		8	8
			%		100.00%	100.00%

Group A: p= 1.000; Group B: p= 0.016

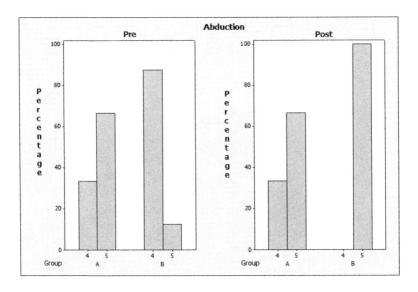

Figure 25 – Percentages for degree of hip abduction muscle strength in groups A and B, pre- and post-treatment

48

Table 13 – Distribution of frequencies and percentages of the degree of hip adduction muscle strength in groups A and B, pre-and post-treatment

GROUP				Post 5	Total
A	Pre	5	Frequency	9	9
			%	100.00%	100.00%
	TOTAL		Frequency	9	9
			%	100.00%	100.00%
B	Pre	4	Frequency	100.00%	100.00%
			%	100.00%	100.00%
		5	Frequency	7	7
			%	100.00%	100.00%
	TOTAL		Frequency	8	8
			%	100.00%	100.00%

Group A: p= 1.000; Group B: p= 1.000

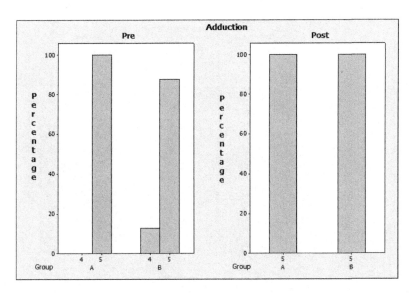

Figure 26 – Percentages for degree of hip adduction muscle strength in groups A and B, pre- and post-treatment

Table 14 – Distribution of frequencies and percentages of the degree of hip medial rotation muscle strength in groups A and B, pre-and post-treatment

GROUP				Post 4	Post 5	Total
A	Pre	4	Frequency	2		2
			%	100.00%		100.00%
		5	Frequency	2	5	7
			%	28.60%	71.40%	100.00%
	TOTAL		Frequency	4	5	9
			%	44.40%	55.60%	100.00%
B	Pre	4	Frequency	4	1	5
			%	80.00%	20.00%	100.00%
		5	Frequency		3	3
			%		100.00%	100.00%
	TOTAL		Frequency	4	4	8
			%	50.00%	50.00%	100.00%

Group A: p= 0.500; Group B: p= 1.000

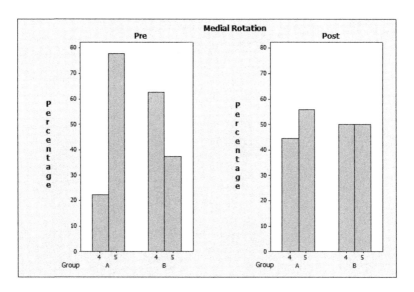

Figure 27 – Percentages for degree of hip medial rotation muscle strength in groups A and B, pre- and post-treatment

Table 15 – Distribution of frequencies and percentages of the degree of hip lateral
rotation muscle strength in groups A and B, pre-and post-treatment

GROUP				Post 4	5	Total
A	Pre	4	Frequency	2		2
			%	100.0%		100.0%
		5	Frequency	1	6	7
			%	14.3%	85.7%	100.0%
	TOTAL		Frequency	3	6	9
			%	33.3%	66.7%	100.0%
B	Pre	4	Frequency	2	1	3
			%	66.7%	33.3%	100.0%
		5	Frequency		5	5
			%		100.0%	100.0%
	TOTAL		Frequency	2	6	8
			%	25.0%	75.0%	100.0%

Group A: p= 1.000; Group B: p= 1.000

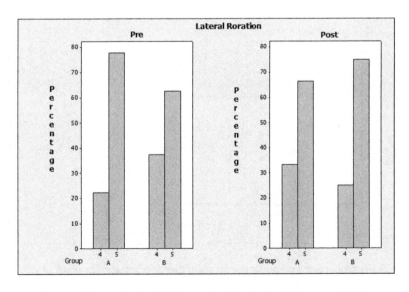

Figure 28 – Percentages for degree of hip lateral rotation muscle strength in groups A and
B, pre- and post-treatment

4.3 Analysis of degree of hip joint dysfunction

Table 16 – Descriptive statistics for degree of hip joint dysfunction by period: pre- and post-treatment and for difference between periods, in groups A and B

	Group	N	Mean	SD	Minimum	Median	Maximum
Pre	A	9	6.3	4.5	1	6	16
	B	8	13.3	4.3	6	14	18
Post	A	9	9.8	4.9	4	9	21
	B	8	3.5	2.1	0	3	7
Pre - Post	A	9	-3.4	1.8	-7	-3	-1
	B	8	9.8	2.7	6	11	13

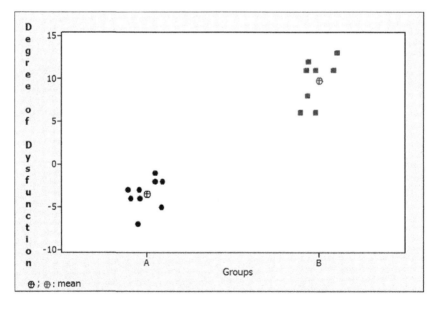

Figure 29 – Individual and mean values for the difference between degrees of joint dysfunction in the pre- and post-treatment periods in groups A and B

Bonferroni Method:

➤ In Group A, the pre-treatment mean is smaller than the post-treatment mean (p<0.001);

➤ In Group B, the pre-treatment mean is larger than the post-treatment mean (p<0.001);

➤ Pre-treatment, the mean for group B is larger than for group A (p≈0.024);

➤ Post-treatment, the mean for group A is larger than for group B (p=0.020).

4.4 Analysis of adherence to treatment in group B

Table 17 – Descriptive statistics for adherence (%) to treatment in group B, by sessions completed

N	Mean	SD	Minimum	Median	Maximum
8	84.38	11.73	70.83	81.25	100.00

5. DISCUSSION OF THE FINDINGS

This chapter comprehends a discussion of the study findings, comparing to other studies published in scientific literature.

Legg-Calvé-Perthes disease (LCPD) was described at the beginning of the last century, in 1910, by Arthur Legg (United States of America), Jacques Calvé (France) and Georg Perthes (Germany), who described and conceptualized it almost simultaneously (Nevelös, 1996).

To the present day, there has been no single theory that explains what leads to the transient obstruction of the femoral head circulation. Among the speculations presented as possible causes: hereditary thrombophilia (Lopez-Franco et al., 2005), increased blood viscosity (Kleimann and Bleck, 1981), endocrine factors (Kealey et al., 2000); increased intracapsular hydrostatic pressure and transient synovitis (Tachdjian, 2001). There are also references to a possibly genetic origin, but no testable pattern of inheritance has been able to be established (Hall et al. 1979; Wynne-Davies, 1980).

The age of patients in both groups was considered statistically equal, averaging 5.6 years for group A and 5.7 years for group B. Martinez et al. (1992) had an average age of six years in their study, while Tsao et al. (1997) found an average age of 4.4 years. Thus, it is considered that the average age in this study showed no differences between groups and no differences with the literature. Age is considered a prognostic factor, the younger the better the prognosis, due to the longer time to remodel until skeletal maturity. Fabry et al. (2003) reported that, generally speaking, the younger, the better the chances of a successful treatment outcome. Successful treatments do not always occur.

The ratio between the number of males to females is consistently described in studies in the literature as 4:1 (Catterall, 1971; Bohr, 1980; Friedlander and Weiner, 2000; Gigante et al., 2002; Guarniero et al., 2005).

In this study, both groups showed similar results regarding the percentage of female patients: 11.1% in group A (one patient) and 12.5% (one patient) in group B. These values diverge somewhat from the literature. However, they are consistent with another study performed in this same Institute, where the proportion of female patients was 9.8% (Guarniero et al., 1997). In contrast with other studies also conducted in similar environments, but in different locations, there were similar proportions of female participants, such as 20% (Laredo Filho et al., 1993) and 33.3% (Volpon et al., 1996). Perhaps there is a lower incidence of disease in female patients at this study site. If there was information on incidence at the national level, would be able to correlate it with the lower incidence presented at this study site, requiring larger samples for such a study. It is known that female patients have a worse prognosis when compared to males, girls reaching skeletal maturity before boys, thus reducing the hip joint remodeling period (Gershuni, 1980; Grzegorzewska et al., 2003).

The predominant race was Caucasian: seven patients (77.8%) in group A and seven patients (87.5%) in group B. In two studies conducted in Brazil, the predominance of Caucasian patients was eight (88.9%) among nine studied (Ishida et al., 1998a). In another study of 43 patients, it was 95.35%, comprising 41 cases (Ishida et al., 1998b). In this sample, it was also noted that despite being statistically equal, the incidence of blacks was higher compared to other studies in Brazil. This could be related to the fact that this study had a small sample. Bohr (1980) emphasizes that the disease is rare in Africa and in the Black population of the United States of America.

According to Wenger et al. (1991), the involvement of the left and right hips is approximately equal in relation to LCPD. In this study, group A showed an impairment in six left hips (66.7%), while in group B, six (75%) of the affected hips were right. In their work, Guille et al. (1998) found equal involvement of the right and left hip in patients with LCPD. The fact that group A showed a larger involvement of the right hip was not considered to make it different from group B. It also does not differentiate it from data in the literature, since even though papers reporting a higher frequency of the left hip have been presented, no statistical difference was found in them. The lack of statistical significance in this study may not implicate a difference between the groups because of the small sample size.

In this study, there was a greater percentage of patients having right side dominance in both groups: five (55.6%) in group A and six (75%) in group B, considered to be statistically equal. No data were found in the literature that relate the affected hip with the dominant side of patients with LCPD.

The diagnosis of LCPD is done by clinical assessment and is confirmed radiographically (Mose, 1980). One of the first symptoms for this evaluation is pain and/or limping. The pain described may be in the hip, but usually refers to the medial thigh or knee (Carpernter, 1975; Laredo Filho et al., 2002). During clinical evaluation, patients with LCPD may also present a positive on the Trendelenburg test (Edvardsen et al., 1981), decreased hip ROM, especially in abduction, flexion and medial rotation, which may lead to hypertrophy or atrophy of the thigh, due to the disuse of the limb (Carpenter, 1975; Laredo Filho et al., 2002), abductor muscle deficiency due to the increased growth of the greater trochanter (Bowen et al., 1982) and flexion and abduction hip muscle contracture

(Sugimoto et al., 2004). Thus, it is important to measure the degree of ROM and hip muscle strength (Carpenter, 1975; Edvardsen et al., 1981, Jacobs et al., 2004; Guarniero et al., 2005), because the results of treatment are directly related to hip ROM. When the patient presents no symptoms and maintains complete hip ROM (Catterall, 1971), it is considered a good treatment outcome. Thus, the decline of hip ROM can be an early sign of a subluxation (Catterall, 1981). In this study, hip ROM for the movements performed showed, on average, a restriction in range of motion. In groups A and B, most of the muscles of the affected hip showed an average loss of strength compared with the unaffected hip. Thus, these data were used to compare the results obtained by the proposed treatments.

To classify the stage and prognosis of the disease, special radiographic classifications were adopted in the literature: Catterall (1971) classified the stages of LCPD according to four types of radiographic findings, depending on the extent of the femoral epiphysis lesion; Salter and Thompson (1984) created a classification based on radiographic signs of subchondral lysis (fracture), divided into two types, A and B; Herring et al. (1992) described a classification based on the height of the lateral pillar of the epiphysis in the fragmentation phase, subdividing the hips into three types: A, B and C. Later, Herring et al. (2004a) adapted the original lateral pillar classification, subdividing it into four types: A, B, B/C and C.

In this study, patients in groups A and B showed a radiographic basis for conservative treatment. Catterall, Salter and Thompson, and Herring classifications were adopted. In group B only, two patients (25%) were found with Catterall type I. Seven patients (77.8%) were found to have Herring type B in group A and five patients (62.5%) in group B. This is probably due to the difficulty of this disease's early diagnosis and the study site being a tertiary hospital, where more complex cases are referred, most often requiring surgical procedures. It was only possible to use the Salter and Thompson classification in four patients (44.4%) in group A and in three patients (37.5%) in group B, since it was not always possible to see the subchondral fracture in radiographs. Wiig et al. (2004) found the subchondral fracture in only 92 patients (23.5%) of their 392 patients.

Some criticize the Catterall classification for its low reproducibility creating inter-observer disagreement (Hardeastle et al. 1980; Mukherjee and Fabry, 1990), and the possibility of change according to disease phase (Van Dam et al. 1981; Mukherjee and Fabry, 1990). The Salter and Thompson classification attempted to solve these problems through a more simple and reproducible system. However, this classification can only be used in the early stages of the disease, when the subchondral fracture is visible, applicable to only a small number of patients (Ritterbusch et al. 1993; Santili et al., 1999). The Herring classification has been widely and successfully used in determining prognosis (Mukherjee and Fabry, 1990; Machado Neto and Dias, 1999). Agus et al. (2004) found that the Catterall and Salter and Thompson classifications should be used to determine the prognosis of the disease. Friedlander and Weiner (2000), however, believed that the Herring classification was very useful for their study. In this study, they sought to minimize such problems by centralizing all comments and radiographic classifications with the same evaluator.

The literature describes the following as the main classifications used for radiographic evaluation of treatment: Mose (1980) reported the need to measure the lesion of the femoral head in LCPD, with the goal of obtaining a prognosis in relation to osteoarthritis of the hip of the patient as an adult; Stulberg et al. (1981) created a radiological classification based on results obtained after treatment of LCPD. This classification should be used when patients have reached skeletal maturity, which divides patients into five groups according to severity of outcome. Agus et al. (2004) believed that the Stulberg classification should be used to sort the treatment results of patients who have reached skeletal maturity, but according to the authors, a dilemma remains regarding how to classify patients who have not yet reached skeletal maturity. Eventually, patients included in this study could be evaluated on the basis of previously described radiographic classifications.

The main goal of treatment is to maintain the best possible hip joint morphology, prevent early degeneration and maintain joint mobility, while providing pain relief (Martinez et al., 1992, Herring et al. 1993; Wang et al., 1995).

Surgical treatment is indicated for patients over the age of six years with Catterall classification type III and IV and/or Herring type B. The surgical procedures most frequently offered to patients with LCPD in Brazil are Salter osteotomy (Salter, 1980; Tachdjian, 2001), proximal varus osteotomy of the femur (Guarniero et al. 1995; Guarniero et al., 1997 ; Friedlander and Weiner, 2000) and hip arthrodiastasis (Luzo, 1998; Volpon et al., 1998).

There are various forms of conservative treatment, and the earlier patients are treated, the better the prognosis (Katz, 1967). According Kitakoji et al. (2005), not all surgical treatments are more indicated than conservative treatments.

Initially, Pike (1950) described the treatment using skin traction for three weeks, then using weight-bearing orthoses with an average of 28 months of hospitalization. With the follow-up for 8 to 12 years, 83% good results were observed. Brotherton and McKibbin

(1977) evaluated patients 17 years after treatment with bed rest and weight-bearing restrictions for 26 months on average and had 88% good and 10% poor results. Thompson and Westin (1979) reported that both the high hospital costs and psychological problems generated by a long period of hospitalization were reasons to shorten the hospitalization period. They demonstrated that when patients are released after a shorter hospital stay for daily activities before there is complete restoration of the femoral head and at the stage of reossification, there is no detriment to treatment outcome.

Petrie and Bitenc in 1971, are the first to introduce the concept of treatment by containment of the femoral head through the creation of an orthesis. They believed that relieving abduction load helped modeling of the femoral head, reducing the irregularities on its surface. According to the authors, the method requires frequent changes of plaster cast, and because knee and ankle restraint is necessary, these joints develop a temporary stiffness. Later, Meehan et al. (1992) developed their hip abduction orthosis, which was a modification of the orthosis developed by Petrie and Bitenc. Meehan et al. (1992) and Martinez et al. (1992) studied the results after the use of abduction orthosis with load relief. In both papers, Stulberg and Mose criteria were used to evaluate the results. No improvement was observed when compared with untreated patients. Thus, the use of abduction orthosis, which was widespread among the 70s and 80s, began to show poor results through retrospective studies, when patients were followed for long periods. In 2000, Weinstein, studying results reported in the literature and the results of his own studies on the use of abduction devices with load relief for the legs, concluded that there was little support for the effectiveness of abduction bracing and no longer recommended it.

Kelly et al. (1980) published their results of patients with unilateral LCPD who were treated with partial weight-bearing relief without any device containing the femoral head. They concluded that when children are classified as Catterall type III or IV early in the disease, they should be treated by femoral head containment methods. The children with lesser involvement of the femoral head may be accompanied with no weight-bearing restriction. Catterall (1980) described how of patients belonging to his classification types I, II and III, under five years of age and with no signs of risk, 60% obtained good results without treatment.

Other studies in the literature show conservative forms of treatment with very different methodologies that apply more than one form of treatment without separating their results. Such treatments include broomstick plaster casts (Denton, 1980), Thomas splint (Yrjönen, 1992), Craig brace and Atlanta brace (Herring et al., 1993).

The role of physical therapy in LCPD is not very clear in the literature, regarding its real benefits to LCPD or when it can be used. Numerous articles mention it only as a preoperative and/or postoperative resource (Jani and Dick, 1980, Ishida et al. 1994; Guarniero et al., 1995, Schmid et al., 2003) or as a form of conservative treatment combined with another modality: skin traction, bracing, plaster cast (Klisic et al., 1980, Bowen et al., 1982, Wang et al. 1995; Futami and Suzuki, 1997; Aksoy et al., 2004) used for patients with LCPD.

Some studies report on the importance of physical therapy in LCPD through exercises for maintaining or gaining hip ROM and decreasing muscle spasms (Herring et al. 1994; Wall, 1999). Carpenter (1975) described the exercises and physical therapy resources that can be used in LCPD, such as active-assisted exercises, active and active-resisted, proprioceptive neuromuscular facilitation (PNF), cryotherapy and hydrotherapy.

Keret et al. (2002) showed the improvement of the ROM and hip pain relief with physical therapy on ground and in water. Felicio et al. (2005) performed physical therapy with exercises to gain hip ROM and gain hip muscle strength in a patient who underwent hip arthrodiastasis while using the device and after removing it, showing significant improvement.

Sposito et al. (1992) studied patients who underwent modified Salter osteotomy and carried out a rehabilitation program after surgery, obtaining better posture. In contrast, patients who did not perform postoperative rehabilitation showed deterioration. Herring et al. (2004b), in one of their treatment groups, performed active exercises to gain hip ROM, finding no statistical difference when compared to other conservative treatments. Carney and Minter (2004) retrospectively studied 118 patients with LCPD and reported that 42 had a gain in hip ROM with several nonsurgical treatments such as physical therapy on ground and in water.

According to Sposito et al. (1992), there were no specific studies in the literature more deeply or broadly addressing the topic of physical therapy for LCPD. Wild et al. (2003) suggested conducting a study with patients with LCPD, with indication for conservative treatment, and undergoing physical therapy for three to four months, monitored by clinical and radiographic evaluations. According to the authors, most articles they studied described the importance of physical therapy in treating the disease. However, the procedures recommended for physical therapy treatment were not described.

For one study group (group A), the treatment recommended in the literature for patients referred for conservative treatment of LCPD was performed, with observation and outpatient follow-up (Catterall, 1980).

Having performed literature search and having not found the physical therapy procedures to be adopted for patients with indication for conservative treatment of LCPD, and whether these procedures would lead to some improvement of hip ROM, muscle strength and the radiographic picture, this study was carried out on these variables to seek answers to these questions. Therefore, and since few studies were found of the disease applied to physical therapy, this program also sought to use means described in the physical therapy literature (Kisner and Colby, 1998; Bandy and Sanders, 2003). Thus, for the other study group (group B), I sought to develop a therapy program based on passive stretching exercises to gain ROM in the affected hip, active strengthening exercises to increase muscle strength in the affected limb, and balance training.

Herring et al. (1994) reported that most studies do not use a control group and are rarely compared with other results and studies. Ten years later, Herring et al. (2004b) reported the existence of only a few controlled studies in the literature and only one randomized study. Thus, we attempted to conduct a prospective controlled inquiry in this study.

Clinical evaluation was based on ROM, the degree of muscle strength and the degree of hip dysfunction (Sposito et al. 1992; Felicio et al., 2005), which are easily reproduced in clinical practice. Patients were observed for any radiographic changes.

Before starting the discussion of the evaluated results, it would be appropriate to clarify the hypotheses originally proposed. In the Introduction of this thesis, two hypotheses were considered. Since there was a statistically significant difference between the means of the groups in this study, the null hypothesis (H0), which considered that there would be no significant difference between group means, was rejected.

In the analysis of ROM of patients in group B, all movements studied showed statistically significant improvement in changes in their average when comparing pre and post-treatment. Group A showed no improvement between pre- and post-treatment. Patients remained the same or worsened ($p = 0.005$ for abduction, $p = 0.050$ for adduction). Patients in group B showed an greater average difference of ROM between the affected and unaffected hip in pre-treatment period compared with group A. Post-treatment, this relationship reversed, with group A having a greater mean difference than group B. Thus, the improvement in ROM of group B patients and worsening of group A becomes clear. In literature reviewed, there are few studies that report the ROM values for after completion of treatment and those that usually reported them showed values for patients who underwent a reassessment years after conservative treatments and surgical treatments were completed. Felicito et al. (2005) studied a patient who initially presented 60 degrees flexion, 0° of extension, 25° of abduction, 10° of adduction, a medial rotation of 5°, and 15° lateral rotation of the hip affected with LCPD. This patient, who was treated with surgery and possibly presented greater impairment than the patients in this study, proved difficult to compare results after treatment.

Since the degree of muscle strength of the unaffected limb was considered grade five in all groups and individuals in both pre- and post-treatment, statistical analysis of the variables of uninvolved limb was not performed. The degree of muscle strength found in patients were equal to four or five, and were considered as such in the statistical analysis. An improvement in the values of the degree of muscle strength in group B was observed in the data regarding degree of muscle strength of the affected hip. The incidence of patients with a post-treatment grade of five was higher than in the pre-treatment for the hip abductor muscles ($p = 0.016$). These were probably the most weakened muscles in pre-treatment. The medial and lateral rotator muscles were also weakened pre-treatment, but strengthening exercises for these muscle groups were not performed in group B. Even so, there was a small, not significant improvement after the stretching exercises. In only a few studies was the degree of muscle strength assessed (Sposito, 1991; Sposito et al., 1992; and Felicio et al., 2005), but it was not possible to compare them with the degree of muscle strength in this study.

The degree of joint dysfunction presented, on average, an improvement in group B and a worsening in group A in relation to the treatment periods. In group A, the mean pre-treatment was lower than in the post-treatment ($p < 0.001$) and group B, the pre-treatment mean was higher than in the post-treatment ($p < 0.001$).

Sposito (1991), in his doctoral dissertation and in a 1992 publication with other authors, established criteria for classifying joint dysfunction, and also creates a classification, based on the score obtained, to characterize the degree of joint dysfunction: seven points, mild; between eight and 20 points, moderate, between 21 and 40 points, severe (Sposito et al., 1992). It is believed that there is great variation among patients so that, for example, someone classified as "moderate" could have a degree of joint dysfunction of eight or even 20, which is a rather large variation in the degree of joint dysfunction. Thus, we opted to not use the classification (mild, moderate or severe) to determine the degree of joint dysfunction, but only the numerical values.

Sposito (1991) found an average pre-treatment level of articular dysfunction: in group I, Catterall type II patients had 8.8, and type III, 22.5 points, in group II, type II patients averaged 18.8, and type III, 16 points. In this study, we obtained an average of 6.3 pre-treatment in group A and 13.3 in group B. This shows that radiographic features do not always correspond to the grade of joint dysfunction, since in this study group B had patients with less radiographic involvement (Catterall type I) and got an average grade of joint dysfunction greater than that of group A. Thus, like group II in Sposito (1991), patients with Catterall type III presented with 16 points, against 18.8 points in patients with Catterall type II. However, the results after treatment can not be compared due to the fact that treatment and times of treatments were very different.

Patients in both study groups showed no change in radiographic features during the implementation of this study.

Group B's adherence to treatment was 84.4% on average. It is believed that adherence is directly linked to the social and economic conditions of patients and guardians, but, taking that into account, the adherence obtained in this study was considered good adherence to the proposed treatment.

The improvement of patients in group B that underwent the proposed physical therapy program was obvious, and the program could be applied to other patients with LCPD for whom conservative treatment is also indicated. Thus, patients who have a hip ROM limitation, loss of hip muscle strength and a limited level of joint dysfunction would benefit from such treatment. Patients in both study groups showed no radiographic change and will be monitored for further analysis, to ascertain whether there is any radiographic change after patients reach skeletal maturity.

Several obstacles were encountered during this study. Finding patients who were indicated for conservative treatment was a problem, probably due to the difficulty of performing early diagnosis. Another aspect is geographical, since patients are often referred from other states to perform the treatment in major urban centers, which precludes proper monitoring and residence during the treatment period. The socio-economic distortions in this country, and, consequently, the challenges of the healthcare system also result in barriers for some patients and guardians, who were unable to complete the proposed treatment or any other form of treatment. Many aspects remain unknown in LCPD, such as the etiology and which treatments are most directly correlated with it. Many treatments are intended to minimize the deformities that are consequences of the disease and do not directly address the question that remains unclear until today.

6. STUDY CONCLUSIONS

- The exercises proposed for Group B patients were effective in both an improving the range of motion as well as increasing the muscle strength of the hip involved when compared with patients in Group A.
- The physical therapy treatment used in group B was effective for patients with LCPD, when conservative treatment is indicated.

7. REFERENCES

Agus H, Kalenderer O, Eryanlmaz G, Ozcalabi IT. Intraobserver and interobserver reliability of Catterall, Herring, Salter-Thompson and Stulberg classification systems in Perthes disease. *J Pediatr Orthop B.* 2004;13(3):166-9.

Aksoy MC, Caglar O, Yazici M, Alpaslan AM. Comparison between braced and non-braced Legg-Calve-Perthes-disease patients: a radiological outcome study. *J Pediatr Orthop B.* 2004;13(3):153-7.

Bandy WD, Sanders B. *Exercício terapêutico: técnicas para intervenção.* Rio de Janeiro: Guanabara Koogan; 2003.

Brech, GC. *Avaliação do tratamento fisioterapêutico da doença de Legg-Calvé-Perthes* [dissertação]. São Paulo: Faculdade de Medicina, Universidade de São Paulo; 2006.

Brech, G.C. Guarnieiro, R. Evaluation of Physiotherapy in the Treatment of Legg-Calvé-perthes disease. *Clinics.* 2006;61(6):521-8.

Bohr HH. On the development and course of Legg-Calve-Perthes disease (LCPD). *Clin Orthop.* 1980;(150):30-5.

Bowen JR, Schreiber FC, Foster BK, Wein BK. Premature femoral neck physeal closure in Perthes' disease. *Clin Orthop.* 1982;(171):24-9.

Brotherton BJ, McKibbin B. Perthes' disease treated by prolonged recumbency and femoral head containment: a long-term appraisal. *J Bone Joint Surg Br.* 1977;59(1):8-14.

Carney BT, Minter CL. Nonsurgical treatment to regain hip abduction motion in Perthes disease: a retrospective review. *South Med J.* 2004;97(5):485-8.

Carpenter BN. Legg-Calve-Perthes disease. *Phys Ther.* 1975;55(3):242-9.

Catterall A. The natural history of Perthes' disease. *J Bone Joint Surg Br.* 1971;53(1):37-53.

Catterall A. Treatment in Legg-Calve-Perthes' disease. *Acta Orthop Belg.* 1980;46(4):431-4.

Catterall A. Legg-Calve-Perthes syndrome. *Clin Orthop.* 1981;(158):41-52.

Denton JR. Experience with Legg-Calve-Perthes disease (LCPD) 1968-1974 at the New York Orthopaedic Hospital. *Clin Orthop.* 1980;(150):36-42.

Dickens DR, Menelaus MB. The assessment of prognosis in Perthes' disease. *J Bone Joint Surg Br.* 1978;60-B(2):189-94.

Edvardsen P, Slordahl J, Svenningsen S. Operative versus conservative treatment of Legg-Calve-Perthes disease. *Acta Orthop Scand.* 1981;52(5):553-9.

Erkula G, Bursal A, Okan E. False profile radiography for the evaluation of Legg-Calve-Perthes disease. *J Pediatr Orthop B.* 2004;13(4):238-43.

Fabry K, Fabry G, Moens P. Legg-Calve-Perthes disease in patients under 5 years of age does not always result in a good outcome. Personal experience and meta-analysis of the literature. *J Pediatr Orthop B.* 2003;12(3):222-7.

Felício RL, Barros ARSB, Volpon JB. Abordagem fisioterapêutica em crianças com doença de Legg-Calvé-Perthes submetidas à instalação do artrodistrador: estudo de caso. *Fisioter Pesqui.* 2005;11(1):37-42.

Friedlander JK, Weiner DS. Radiographic results of proximal femoral varus osteotomy in Legg-Calve-Perthes disease. *J Pediatr Orthop.* 2000;20(5):566-71.

Futami T, Suzuki S. Different methods of treatment related to the bilateral occurrence of Perthes' disease. *J Bone Joint Surg Br.* 1997;79(6):979-82.

Gershuni DH. Preliminary evaluation and prognosis in Legg-Calve-Perthes disease. *Clin Orthop.* 1980;(150):16-22.

Gigante C, Frizziero P, Turra S. Prognostic value of Catterall and Herring classification in Legg-Calve-Perthes disease: follow-up to skeletal maturity of 32 patients. *J Pediatr Orthop.* 2002;22(3):345-9.

Grzegorzewski A, Bowen JR, Guille JT, Glutting J. Treatment of the collapsed femoral head by containment in Legg-Calve-Perthes disease. *J Pediatr Orthop.* 2003;23(1):15-9.

Grzegorzewski A, Synder M, Kozlowski P, Szymczak W, Bowen RJ. Leg length discrepancy in Legg-Calve-Perthes disease. *J Pediatr Orthop.* 2005;25(2):206-9.

Guarniero R, Luzo CAM, Wlastemir GL, Lage LAA, Iacovone M. A queilectomia como operação de salvamento na patologia do quadril: resultados preliminares. *Rev Bras Ortop.* 1995;30(1-2):42-4.

Guarniero R, Ishikawa MT, Luzo CAM, Montenegro NB, Godoy RM. Resultados da osteotomia femoral varizante no tratamento da doença de Legg-Calvé-Perthes (DLCP). *Rev Hosp Clin Fac Med São Paulo.* 1997;52(3):132-5.

Guarniero R, Andrusaitis FR, Brech GC, Eyherabide AP, Godoi Júnior RM. A avaliação inicial em pacientes com doença de Legg-Calvé-Perthes internados. *Acta Ortop Bras.* 2005;13(2):68-70.

Guille JT, Lipton GE, Szoke G, Bowen JR, Harcke HT, Glutting JJ. Legg-Calve-Perthes disease in girls. A comparison of the results with those seen in boys. *J Bone Joint Surg Am.* 1998;80(9):1256-63.

Hall DJ, Harrison MH, Burwell RG. Congenital abnormalities and Perthes' disease. Clinical evidence that children with Perthes' disease may have a major congenital defect. *J Bone Joint Surg Br.* 1979;61(1):18-25.

Hardeatle PH, Ross R, Hamalainen M, Mata A. Catterall grouping of Perthes disease. An assessment of observer error and prognostic using Catterall classification. *J Bone Joint Surg Br.* 1980;62:428-31.

Herring JA, Neustadt JB, Williams JJ, Early JS, Browne RH. The lateral pillar classification of Legg-Calve-Perthes disease. *J Pediatr Orthop.* 1992;12(2):143-50.

Herring JA, Williams JJ, Neustadt JN, Early JS. Evolution of femoral head deformity during the healing phase of Legg-Calve-Perthes disease. *J Pediatr Orthop.* 1993;13(1):41-5.

Herring JA. The treatment of Legg-Calve-Perthes disease. A critical review of the literature. *J Bone Joint Surg Am.* 1994;76(3):448-58.

Herring JA, Kim HT, Browne R. Legg-Calve-Perthes disease. Part I: Classification of radiographs with use of the modified lateral pillar and Stulberg classifications. *J Bone Joint Surg Am.* 2004a;86(10):2103-20.

Herring JA, Kim HT, Browne R. Legg-Calve-Perthes disease. Part II: Prospective multicenter study of the effect of treatment on outcome. *J Bone Joint Surg Am.* 2004b;86(10):2121-34.

Hoppenfeld S. *Propedêutica ortopédica: coluna e extremidades.* São Paulo: Atheneu; 1999.

Ishida A, Laredo Filho J, Kuwajima SS, Milani C, Pinto JÁ. Osteotomia de Salter no tratamento da doença de Legg-Calvé-Perthes: fixação com pinos rosqueados e não utilização de imobilização gessada. *Rev Bras Ortop.* 1994;29(9):665-9.

Ishida A, Kuwajima SS, Milani C, Adames MK, Benbassat JR. Osteotomia de Chiari na doença de Perthes. *Rev Bras Ortop.* 1998a;33(1):1-7.

Ishida A, Laredo Filho J, Kuwajima SS, Milani C. Avaliação da esfericidade da cabeça femoral pelo método de Mose, em pacientes portadores da doença de Legg-Calvé-Perthes, submetidos à osteotomia de Salter. *Rev Bras Ortop.* 1998b;33(8):637-44.

Jacobs R, Moens P, Fabry G. Lateral shelf acetabuloplasty in the early stage of Legg-Calve-Perthes disease with special emphasis on the remaining growth of the acetabulum: a preliminary report. *J Pediatr Orthop B.* 2004;13(1):21-8.

Jani LF, Dick W. Results of three different therapeutic groups in Perthes' disease. *Clin Orthop.* 1980;(150):88-94.

Joseph B, Varghese G, Mulpuri K, Narasimha Rao KL, Nair NS. Natural evolution of Perthes disease: a study of 610 children under 12 years of age at disease onset. *J Pediatr Orthop.* 2003;23(5):590-600.

Katz JF. Conservative treatment of Legg-Calve-Perthes disease. *J Bone Joint Surg Am.* 1967;49(6):1043-51.

Kealey WD, Moore AJ, Cook S, Cosgrove AP. Deprivation, urbanisation and Perthes' disease in Northern Ireland. *J Bone Joint Surg Br.* 2000;82(2):167-71.

Kelly FB Jr, Canale ST, Jones RR. Legg-Calve-Perthes disease. Long-term evaluation of non-containment treatment. *J Bone Joint Surg Am.* 1980;62(3):400-7.

Kendall FP, McCreary EK, Provance PG. *Músculos: provas e funções.* 4ª ed. São Paulo: Manole; 1995.

Keret D, Lokiec F, Hayek S, Segev E, Ezra E. Perthes-like changes in geleophysic dysplasia. *J Pediatr Orthop B.* 2002;11(2):100-3.

Kisner C, Colby LA. *Exercícios terapêuticos: fundamentos e técnicas.* São Paulo: Manole; 1998.

Kitakoji T, Hattori T, Kitoh H, Katoh M, Ishiguro N. Which is a better method for Perthes' disease: femoral varus or Salter osteotomy? *Clin Orthop.* 2005;(430):163-70.

Kleinman RG, Bleck EE. Increased blood viscosity in patients with Legg-Perthes disease: a preliminary report. *J Pediatr Orthop.* 1981;1(2):131-6.

Klisic P, Blazevic U, Seferovic O. Approach to treatment of Legg-Calve-Perthes disease. *Clin Orthop.* 1980;(150):54-9.

Laredo Filho J, Ishida A, Milani C, Lourenço AF, Kuwajima SS, Jorge SRN. Avaliação radiográfica da cobertura acetabular da cabeça femoral em pacientes portadores da doença de Legg-Calvé-Perthes unilateral submetidos à osteotomia de Salter. *Rev Bras Ortop.* 1993;28(5):299-303.

Laredo Filho J, Ishida A, Milani C, Kuwajima SS. Doença de Legg-Calvé-Perthes. *Diagn tratamento*. 2002;7(1):29-33.

Lecuire F. The long-term outcome of primary osteochondritis of the hip (Legg-Calve-Perthes' disease). *J Bone Joint Surg Br*. 2002;84(5):636-40.

Lopez-Franco M, Gonzalez-Moran G, De Lucas JC Jr, Llamas P, de Velasco JF, Vivancos JC, et al. Legg-perthes disease and heritable thrombophilia. *J Pediatr Orthop*. 2005;25(4):456-9.

Luzo CAM. *Artrodiástase com fixador externo unilateral no tratamento da doença de Legg-Calvé-Perthes* [tese]. São Paulo: Faculdade de Medicina, Universidade de São Paulo; 1998.

Machado Neto L, Dias L. O uso da cintilografia óssea na doença de Perthes. *Rev Bras Ortop*. 1999;34(1):14-20.

Marques AP. *Manual de goniometria*. São Paulo: Manole; 1997.

Martinez AG, Weinstein SL, Dietz FR. The weight-bearing abduction brace for the treatment of Legg-Perthes disease. *J Bone Joint Surg Am*. 1992;74(1):12-21.

Maxwell SL, Lappin KJ, Kealey WD, McDowell BC, Cosgrove AP. Arthrodiastasis in Perthes' disease. Preliminary results. *J Bone Joint Surg Br*. 2004;86(2):244-50.

Meehan PL, Angel D, Nelson JM. The Scottish Rite abduction orthosis for the treatment of Legg-Perthes disease. A radiographic analysis. *J Bone Joint Surg Am*. 1992;74(1):2-12.

Mose K. Methods of measuring in Legg-Calve-Perthes disease with special regard to the prognosis. *Clin Orthop*. 1980;(150):103-9.

Mukherjee A, Fabry G. Evaluation of the prognostic indices in Legg-Calve-Perthes disease: statistical analysis of 116 hips. *J Pediatr Orthop*. 1990;10(2):153-8.

Neter J, Kutner MH, Nachtsheim CJ, Wasserman W. *Applied linear statistical models*. 4ª ed. Chicago: Irwin; 1996.

Nevelös AB. Perthes' disease the family tree. *Clin Orthop*. 1996;(209):13-22.

Petrie JG, Bitenc I. The abduction weight-bearing treatment in Legg-Perthes' disease. *J Bone Joint Surg Br*. 1971;53(1):54-62.

Pike MM. Legg-Perthes disease: a method of conservative treatment. *J Bone Joint Surg Am*. 1950;32-A(3):663-70.

Ritterbusch JF, Shantharam SS, Gelinas C. Comparison of lateral pillar classification and Catterall classification of Legg-Calve-Perthes disease. *J Pediatr Orthop*. 1993;13(2):200-2.

Rowe SM, Chung JY, Moon ES, Jung ST, Lee HJ, Lee JJ. The effects of subluxation of the femoral head with avascular necrosis in growing rabbits. *J Pediatr Orthop*. 2004;24(6):645-50.

Roy DR. Arthroscopic findings of the hip in new onset hip pain in adolescents with previous Legg-Calve-Perthes disease. *J Pediatr Orthop B*. 2005;14(3):151-5.

Salter RB. Legg-Perthes disease: the scientific basis for the methods of treatment and their indications. *Clin Orthop*. 1980;(150):8-11.

Salter RB, Thompson GH. Legg-Calve-Perthes disease. The prognostic significance of the subchondral fracture and a two-group classification of the femoral head involvement. *J Bone Joint Surg Am*. 1984;66(4):479-89.

Santili C, Milani JL, Pinilla NR. Doença de Legg-Calvé-Perthes: análise crítica da classificação de Salter-Thompson. *Rev Bras Ortop*. 1999;34(7):409-14.

Schmid OA, Hemmer S, Wunsche P, Hirschfelder H. The adult hip after femoral varus osteotomy in patients with unilateral Legg-Calve-Perthes disease. *J Pediatr Orthop B*. 2003;12(1):33-7.

Segev E, Ezra E, Wientroub S, Yaniv M. Treatment of severe late onset Perthes' disease with soft tissue release and articulated hip distraction: early results. *J Pediatr Orthop B.* 2004;13(3):158-65.

Spósito MMM. *O valor da reabilitação no tratamento de pacientes portadores da doença de Legg-Calvé-Perthes submetidos à osteotomia de Salter modificada* [tese]. São Paulo: Escola Paulista de Medicina, Universidade Federal de São Paulo; 1991.

Spósito MMM, Masiero D, Laredo Filho J. O valor da reabilitação no tratamento de pacientes portadores da doença de Legg-Calvé-Perthes submetidos à osteotomia de Salter modificada. *Folha méd(BR).* 1992;104(1/2):19-24.

Stulberg SD, Cooperman DR, Wallensten R. The natural history of Legg-Calve-Perthes disease. *J Bone Joint Surg Am.* 1981;63(7):1095-108.

Sugimoto Y, Akazawa H, Miyake Y, Mitani S, Asaumi K, Aoki K, et al. A new scoring system for Perthes' disease based on combined lateral and posterior pillar classifications. *J Bone Joint Surg Br.* 2004;86(6):887-91.

Tachdjian MO. *Ortopedia pediátrica: diagnóstico e tratamento.* Rio de Janeiro: Revinter; 2001.

Thompson GH, Westin GW. Legg-Calve-Perthes disease: Results of discontinuing treatment in the early reossification phase. *Clin Orthop.* 1979;(139):70-80.

Tsao AK, Dias LS, Conway JJ, Straka P. The prognostic value and significance of serial bone scintigraphy in Legg-Calve-Perthes disease. *J Pediatr Orthop.* 1997;17(2):230-9.

Van Dam BE, Crider RJ, Noyes JD, Larsen LJ. Determination of the Catterall classification in Legg-Calve-Perthes disease. *J Bone Joint Surg Am.* 1981;63(6):906-14.

Volpon JB, Bortolin PH, Pagnano RG. Estatura na doença de Legg-Calvé-Perthes. *Rev Bras Ortop.* 1996;31(1):36-40.

Volpon JB, Lima RS, Schimano AC. Tratamento da forma ativa da doença de Legg-Calvé-Perthes pela artrodiástase. *Rev Bras Ortop.* 1998;33(1):8-14.

Wall EJ. Legg-Calve-Perthes' disease. *Curr Opin Pediatr.* 1999;11(1):76-9.

Wang L, Bowen JR, Puniak MA, Guille JT, Glutting J. An evaluation of various methods of treatment for Legg-Calve-Perthes disease. *Clin Orthop.* 1995;(314):225-33.

Weinstein SL. Bristol-Myers Squibb/Zimmer award for distinguished achievement in orthopaedic research. Long-term follow-up of pediatric orthopaedic conditions. Natural history and outcomes of treatment. *J Bone Joint Surg Am.* 2000;82(7):980-90.

Wenger DR, Ward WT, Herring JA. Legg-Calve-Perthes disease. *J Bone Joint Surg Am.* 1991;73(5):778-88.

Westhoff B, Petermann A, Jäger M, Krauspe R. Movement patterns in frontal plane in Legg-Calvé-Perthes disease. *Gait Posture.* 2004;20(suppl):64.

Wiig O, Svenningsen S, Terjesen T. Evaluation of the subchondral fracture in predicting the extent of femoral head necrosis in Perthes disease: a prospective study of 92 patients. *J Pediatr Orthop B.* 2004;13(5):293-8.

Wild A, Westhoff B, Raab P, Krauspe R. Die nichtoperative therapie des morbus Perthes. *Orthopäde.* 2003;32(2):139-45.

Wynne-Davies R. Some etiologic factors in Perthes' disease. *Clin Orthop.* 1980;(150):12-5.

Yrjonen T. Prognosis in Perthes' disease after noncontainment treatment. 106 hips followed for 28-47 years. *Acta Orthop Scand.* 1992;63(5):523-6.

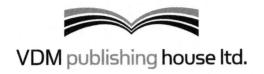
 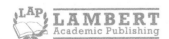 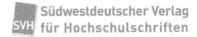

Printed in Great Britain
by Amazon

34324149R00046